# Naturally Healing HERBS

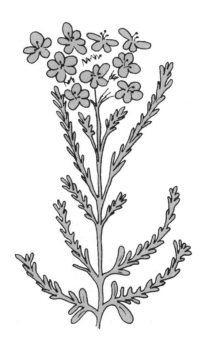

## Carly Wall

**STERLING PUBLISHING CO., INC.**
NEW YORK

Edited by Jeanette Green
Photography by Amy Bridge

**Library of Congress Cataloging-in-Publication Data**

Wall, Carly, 1960–
  Naturally healing herbs / by Carly Wall.
     p.     cm.
  Includes index.
  ISBN 0-8069-3801-3
  1. Herbs—Therapeutic use.   2. Tonics (Medicinal preparations)
I. Title.
RM666.H33W325     1996                                        95-52378
615'.321—dc20


                    1   3   5   7   9   10   8   6   4   2

                Published by Sterling Publishing Company, Inc.
                387 Park Avenue South, New York, N.Y. 10016
                            © 1996 by Carly Wall
                    Distributed in Canada by Sterling Publishing
            % Canadian Manda Group, One Atlantic Avenue, Suite 105
                        Toronto, Ontario, Canada M6K 3E7
                Distributed in Great Britain and Europe by Cassell PLC
                Wellington House, 125 Strand, London WC2R 0BB, England
                Distributed in Australia by Capricorn Link (Australia) Pty Ltd.
        P.O. Box 6651, Baulkham Hills, Business Centre, NSW 2153, Australia
                    *Manufactured in the United States of America*
                            *All rights reserved*

                        Sterling ISBN 0-8069-3801-3

The cover photo of echinacea (the purple cone flower) is by Amy Bridge.

Observe all cautions outlined in this book, and consult a physician before undergoing a tonic regimen. Herbal tonics should not be considered substitutes for medical advice and care that only a physician can provide.

# Contents

‹∂›

# Introduction

To cleanse and renew, that's what we hope for, that's what we search for. Like others before him, Juan Ponce de León set out in 1513 in search for the Fountain of Youth, a legendary spring reported to rejuvenate the body and banish old age. What he found instead was Florida. But de León's failure has not deterred us from our search. We chase after dreams of recapturing lost youth and regaining health and strength. As we age, we try this cream and that exercise program, all to no avail. And we still wonder whether something out there will really work.

Sickness, it seems, goes hand-in-hand with aging. Our bodies have a built-in renewal system, especially when we're young. Just watch a child to see how quickly he or she bounces back from an illness. But as we age, it becomes harder and harder to bounce back. Somehow our body's renewal system goes haywire. If we were to capture the elusive dream of eternal youth and eternal renewal, it would mean discovering how to help heal the body through our own self-defense system, the immune system. We'd love to find a drink so packed with vitamins and minerals and everything the body needs that it could nourish the body into super health. I believe herbal tonics are the answer for our fountain of youth. Let's explore why.

Disease, scientists affirm, has been with us practically since the beginning of human life. And very early humans likely turned to plants to help ease their misery. According to historical records, Mesopotamian, Egyptian, Greek, and Roman physicians all turned to healing plants to cleanse and renew the body and fight disease. Druid priests and healers, who also studied astrology and divination, believed that both plants and humans were affected by the moon's cycles. Barbara Griggs in *Green Pharmacy: The History & Evolution of Western Herbal Medicine* (1991) states that they valued wood betony, feverwort, and vervain, among other herbs, some of which were also prized by ancient Greeks and Romans.

Virtually every culture from Africa to Europe, Asia, Australia, the Americas, and many islands in between has used some form of herbal healing. We marvel at how the earliest healers learned which plant was helpful and which harmful. Perhaps it was by trial and error—observing the patient's reactions. Had the patient been lucky, he survived, and maybe the illness disappeared. But another method may have been used by some healers. When humans lived close to nature, perhaps they possessed a more instinctive ability to choose plants which could be helpful and to avoid plants which could be dangerous. Griggs suggests that "medicinal use of plants seems to have been based on a highly developed 'dowsing' instinct, which led the healer of the tribe to the right plant and taught him or her its use." Today, since we have divorced ourselves from the natural world, this seems strange. Perhaps we have lost an ability we once had.

However, we can often tell if a plant is poisonous by the awful smell or scary appearance it presents. We just need to take time to observe it. But is it so farfetched that we could tell, through instinct, which plants heal certain ills? Paracelsus's (1493–1541) once popular doctrine of signatures asserts that "like heals like" and links plants and their physical character-istics with illnesses humans wish to treat. Under this theory, plants with yellow flowers, say, were thought good for liver problems, and plants with red spots or red flowers were supposed helpful for blood disorders. Amaz-ingly, studies today have supported some of these herbal uses.

In Africa a species of ironweed, *Veronia amygdalina*, contains strong antibiotic and antiparasitic substances. African healers have regularly used its leaves, roots, and bark to treat many illnesses, such as stomach disorders, malaria, and rheumatism. Recently, Michael Huffman, a prima-tologist at Kyoto University in Japan, traveled to Africa to observe chimpan-zees. He noticed one chimp who seemed tired, had diarrhea, and would not eat with the rest of the group. He watched in surprise while the sick chimp searched and found a certain plant, the same *Veronia amygdalina*, and chewed on it. Native shamans favored this plant, which was rarely consumed by chimpanzees. The sick chimp stripped the bark and leaves from a tender branch, chewed it, and drank the juice, then spat out the fiber. The next day, the chimp was back to normal. Huffman and a growing number of researchers have been observing bears, chimpanzees, and other animals that medicate themselves by using the plants around them as their pharmacy.

Some scientists have begun to observe animals in the hope of finding new drugs to cure dreaded ills from plants undiscovered in deep forests. This new field of study is called zoopharmacognosy (discovery of natural drugs by observing animals).

Many herbalists have postulated that for every disease a plant can be found somewhere to cure it. That's why threats to our rain forests and natural environment may also threaten our own healthy existence.

Recipes for Essiac tonic, Hoxsey's Cure, and other herbal remedies have been carefully passed from family to family and friend to friend. These mixtures have helped women with breast cancer, reduced tumors, and regenerated the immune systems of terminal patients. None of these herbal remedies can claim to save all patients, but conventional medicines fail to match their potency. In John Kairns's study at Harvard University, chemo-therapy was found to benefit only 5 percent of cancer patients, although this form of therapy is routinely given to 50 percent of all American cancer sufferers. Herbs used in herbal remedies for cancer and other illnesses are proven blood cleansers that usually strengthen the immune system and serve as a liver tonic as well.

Plant medicinals are simple, inexpensive, and easy to prepare in your own home. However, they have gotten some bad press, and we have been led to believe, falsely, that they're either dangerous or ineffective. It is time these falsehoods are replaced with facts. Both conventional medicine and alternative health care are valuable, and each has its place. Let's hope that in the future both can work side by side to bring about good health to patients who seek it. In the meantime, we can learn as much as we can about alternative health care and, indeed, perhaps even *prevent* illness by keeping our bodies strong. Prevention is the key in herbal healing.

We can see how important this is when we realize that our antibiotics are no longer as effective as they once were. Epidemics, pandemics, and killers like AIDS and cancer threaten us and our loved ones. New diseases seem to be cropping up all over as well as new strains of old illnesses we once thought conquered. Our bodies act as a fort holding out against these invaders. It only makes sense that we have to work to build ourselves up. Look at the stresses we have to contend with: pesticides, pollution, food additives, and ozone depletion, as well as our harried, modern life style. Many people are returning to the natural world, to our roots, as it were, for answers.

## GETTING TO THE ROOT OF THE MATTER

Many early tribes in North America used a certain imposing tree with an oily, highly fragrant bark to make a tea from its leaves and roots. The brew was thought to cure many illnesses, even the plague. Legend has it that this tree, which we know as sassafras, even lured Columbus with its heady scent to find the New World. The tree provided one of the most important medicines for early American tribes. After the Colonists landed, native tribes shared their knowledge of what some called the miracle tree. Thousands of pounds of sassafras roots and leaves were soon exported all over the world.

For generations, farmers in late winter dug fragrant sassafras roots, carefully scrapping off the outer covering, and cleaning and drying them. These roots, an important part of a spring ritual, were guarded. In early spring bits of the root were boiled to make a tea. Families gathered around the stove to enjoy the sweet, sharp smell. Although the outdoor world was still gloomy and muddy, the smell of sassafras roots quickened the pulse. This spring tonic reportedly could "thin the blood and get one ready for all the activities after a winter spent sitting before a fire." Sassafras tonic was said to reduce fevers, relieve weak stomachs and indigestion, heal scurvy and syphilis, and reduce symptoms of menopause. It was also used as a dressing for wounds.

The Pacific yew tree, which is relatively rare, has been found to contain taxol, a chemical used to treat ovarian cancer. This fact known, patients and physicians clamored so much for this tree that it had to be protected. An extract from a creeping vine inhabiting the Cameroon rain forest has been reported to inhibit the replication of the AIDS virus. And the kudzu vine seems to be a wonder plant since it appears to prevent alcohol cravings in alcoholics.

In *Dr. Wright's Guide to Healing with Nutrition* (1990), widely read medical columnist Dr. Jonathon Wright states, "Researchers have also pointed a finger at the pasteurization of milk; the relative lack of zinc . . . and other minerals . . . the intentional addition of food chemicals; and even the unintentional additions of insecticides, pesticides, industrial chemicals, and toxic minerals as the cause of much disease in 'civilized' areas of the world." In 1973 in Michigan a few hundred pounds of polybrominated biphenyls (PBBs) were accidentally mixed into animal feed, which meant that thousands of cattle, sheep, and hogs and millions of chickens died or had to be slaughtered. But about 9 million Michigan residents consumed PBB-tainted meat or dairy products. By 1976, the chemical was still found in mothers' milk. In one Michigan study, 18 of the 45 residents exposed demonstrated seriously defective immune-system functions. The other 27 also demonstrated some type of change, but in a lesser degree. When there is a combination of nutritional deficiency and chemical contamination, you can usually bet on disease.

We need to understand the plants themselves to understand how they heal. Here we delve into pharmacognosy, a field in which scientists attempt to study and identify chemicals and molecules occurring in plants which can be applied medicinally. In the 19th century most medicines—about 80 percent—were made from plants. As time passed, pharmaceutical companies formed and, with them, more sophisticated methods for discovering and isolating active properties contained within living plants. Today, only a quarter of prescription drugs in the United States actually contain a compound derived from plants. Synthetic chemicals created in laboratories are easier and cheaper to manufacture. Also, the drug industry does not have to grow and gather plants. In labs chemicals are isolated and concentrated, while in nature plants combine various chemicals which create a healing blend. Chemical synthetics have caused side effects and other problems many plants, used whole, do not. Inside the human body and inside the plant itself, healing takes place gently, naturally. Many chemical synthetics, instead of removing the cause of the disease or the disease itself, merely mask or suppress symptoms. They function like many over-the-counter cold or flu remedies by, for example, reducing nasal congestion but not shortening the duration of the illness.

Botanists have estimated that only 10 percent of the flowering plant species have been investigated for medical use. Although plant-derived products account for more than $5 billion in medical sales in the United States, for instance, it has been estimated that only 4 percent of the world's plants have been analyzed for pharmacological use. That leaves over a million species of plant as yet unexplored. Simply consider the plants we call weeds because we do not know what's contained inside their leaves, stems, flowers, berries, and roots.

We've fallen very far from the tree, since we have been so caught up with our own inventions in a complicated technical and industrial world. Few people grow their own food anymore. Most of us buy our foods at groceries and some of us eat prepared foods from restaurants and delicatessens. These foods are often subject to bacteria, chemical sprays, and radiation. Produce is often painted and waxed so that no one can guess its age. And many processed foods are chemical-laden creations with little or no remaining nutritive value. Also, many foods grown on small private farms as well as on corporate farms are raised in nutrient-poor soil. Our lands have been raped, sprayed, and used up.

But we've been relearning old methods for renewing dead soils by mulching and composting. We've also been rediscovering many plants that are available to help us build and revitalize our bodies and our health. Plants are packed with nutrition and healing, life-renewing juices.

## WHAT ARE TONICS?

Herbs in ointments, tinctures, extracts, syrups, and drinks have been used to heal in various ways. Each herb considered in this book has certain healing properties for diseases the body may struggle with, like colds, flus, infections, or ulcers. Herbs with properties that prevent disease are called tonic herbs. A *tonic* is a medicinal preparation used to restore tone and vigor to the body for people apparently suffering from a deficiency. These tonics are formulated to relieve certain symptoms, like malaise, lethargy, and loss of appetite, as well as the varied effects of stress, like headaches, insomnia, stomach disorders, and nervousness. Tonics are herbal extracts that contain high vitamin and mineral content designed to strengthen and purify the body and to improve the immune system. In this sense, a tonic is not really a medicine. It's a healthful brew designed to invigorate the body so that it can fight disease. The fact that these tonics cure devastating illnesses and relieve minor discomforts is merely a magical side effect. These tonic drinks are usually strong herbal teas or infusions. For centuries people have used single herbs, but tonics also contain a combination of several herbs. In the 19th century, no one would have thought twice about digging up an herb from the backyard or drinking an herbal pick-me-up at the local drugstore when needed. Today much plant knowledge has almost been forgotten.

This book can help you discover ways to use herbs in tonic form to regenerate, renew, and cleanse your body of the many toxins we encounter today. Herbs can help you become and stay healthy in a natural way. All you need to do is become acquainted with appropriate herbal tonics.

## TONICS AND WHAT THEY DO

We need to have strong bodies if we are to have healthy bodies. You cannot trade in your run-down body for a newer model after you've abused and used up your old body. Life isn't much fun when you're broken down and ill. Many view good health as the natural state; it's only when our bodies are out of balance that illness arrives.

What could be more natural than the plants growing around us which have proven healing properties? Dr. Linda Rector-Page in *How to Be Your Own Herbal Pharmacist* (1994) states, "As medicine, herbs are essentially body balancers that work with the body functions" so that the body can "heal and regulate itself." Tonics are herbs found to help the body do this work itself. They can break up toxins and flush them from body tissues, tone organs, and restore balance to a body that has been neglected and misused.

Many herbalists stress that healing is a slow occurrence that demands a turn-around period of at least 1 month for every year of sickness. One sign when taking an herbal tonic is an actual worsening of the condition, which then allows remarkable healing. In herbal circles it's referred to as the "law of the cure." This worsening occurs when the body begins to throw off toxins and wastes. We conventionally say you "feel worse before getting better." People who have taken Essiac report vomiting and diarrhea that sometimes lasts several days. After this period, the path ahead seems brighter.

But not everyone experiences such seemingly miraculous cures. Every *body* is different. Biochemist and nutritionist Roger Williams, who discovered some of the B vitamins, insists on our "biochemical individuality." And there are times when the immune system is simply too weakened to rebuild. However, it does not hurt to try, and sometimes results can be incredible.

The road to feeling the best we can is open to all of us. Herbs are a gentle means of transportation. Unlike other medicines or vitamins, it's hard to overdo use of herbs. Herbs work on balancing the body since they contain the many different chemicals that work together in a healthful, balanced

10

way. If we do not need a certain substance contained in the herb, the body naturally flushes it out. That's why it does not hurt even to take a strong tonic like Essiac even if you have no signs of cancer. It will help the body if it needs to be helped. Otherwise, the tonic will do little more than help cleanse the body. And if the body is already cleansed and renewed, you'll simply pass the tonic and that will be that.

If you have suffered the effects of modern life—stress, overload, sluggishness, sleeping difficulties, and feeling generally run-down and old—then perhaps you need a tonic to flush out all the toxins you've accumulated. A good tonic could prevent future health difficulties. If your health problems are more severe, you desperately need a tonic to boost your immune system and to help your body return to its natural healthy state. Of course, you should consult a physician before changing your diet or taking any herbal tonics. Also, be sure to follow your physician's instructions concerning health care. These herbal tonics should be merely an addition to any health-care program. Herbal tonics are nature's way of feeding the body back to good health.

If you're looking for a fountain of youth, herbal tonics probably provide the closest thing. If you'd like to embark on a healing path easy to follow, these tonics are the ticket. In this book I've posted a few guidelines to help you on the way.

# History of Tonics

Humans and plants have always been intertwined. To understand the history of tonics, let's begin with the Middle Ages, when a correlation between herbal healing and spirituality or religion reemerged. The climate of medieval Europe included tragic outbreaks of plagues, periodic famines, lawlessness, declining populations, abandoned villages, peasant uprisings, falling agrarian prices, and the misery of drawn-out wars. After the fall of the Roman Empire, religious hermits, who shut themselves away from society, had begun devoting their lives to God.

Eventually, small bands of believers began to form and Christian monasteries developed. Many early monks wished to live simply in solitude and to spend their lives in quiet contemplation. For these colonies of monks to survive, gardens had to be cared for and bees cultivated, and all food, medicines, and other basics had to be fashioned by the monks' own industry, thereby allowing them to remain independent of the outside world. As religious orders were created, they combined simplicity, quiet, and study with a consuming love of gardening. The first medicinal gardens of this battered medieval Europe were sown in early monasteries. Usually monks tended three gardens: the kitchen garden, the orchard and vineyard, and the physic garden full of useful healing herbs.

As Christianity slowly spread throughout Europe, so did the idea of religious community life. The first European monastic gardens had been described in detail in the early 11th century. Before this time, we have only bits and pieces of art or ruins to supply historical hints. Since many communities required protection from enemies and thieves, walls were erected around them. Many monastic and feudal communities became almost citylike and most were self-sustaining. They contained gardens for food, medicines, and flowers, as well as mills, moats, and ponds for fish. So, people within these walled monasteries enjoyed protection, healthy food, and religious conviction.

But few knew how to read or write, and superstition was rampant. Some believed in evil spirits, others were frightened by witchcraft, and many relied on priest-healers, the monks themselves, when sick. And in these early centuries, many epidemics and plagues were prevalent.

Many monks, the learned men of their time, turned a gardening pastime into a passion. Many monasteries maintained a network between the different orders that allowed them to exchange messages and seeds. Also, many monks, unlike some reclusive brothers, traveled freely. Some discovered ancient Greek and other manuscripts written by wise old healers, which they translated, copied, and passed on to other monks and other monasteries. These scholarly monks can be credited for the survival of this ancient wisdom, which they cherished and protected. The monks themselves did not add much new wisdom, however. The founder of the monastery Vivarium in southern Italy edited and translated medical texts and encouraged his disciples to study medicine. He also cared for the sick within the monastery. His high standards within the scriptoria, where monks copied manuscripts, were emulated by other monastic communities.

But these same monastic communities were divided about caring for the sick. Since they could make money from the sale of medicinal herbs and this sale often involved contact with the outside world, some religious leaders forbade monks to practice medicine. But in England, this command was pretty much ignored; there, in the 12th century, monasteries were the only places one could receive medical help or find medical books. By the end of the 13th century, many English abbeys were busily tending the destitute sick. This care for the sick and aged was most considerate, spacious infirmaries often being located apart from the monks' quarters. Infirmaries were well equipped with a pharmacy, kitchen, and large fireplace. Some even had individual cells for patients.

Herb-tending monks were in charge of healing, since physicians were only employed within the most populous abbeys. Faricius, an Italian physician and abbot of Abingdon (from 1100 to 1117), a Benedictine abbey in England, became famous for his abilities. He served as court healer to Henry I and Queen Matilda of England, and to baronial families. Four monk physicians tended the ill at St. Albans, a Benedictine abbey in southern England, from 1183 to 1195. Orval, a famous pharmacy in what is today Luxembourg, was run by the monk Antoine Périn from the mid- to late 1700s. Brother Périn, who had been trained in Paris as a physician, grew many of the roots, herbs, and flowers he needed in a tidy monastic garden. His most popular products were potions and tinctures. The tonic Water of Orval was believed to be effective against a wide variety of ills, both physical and mental. Its fame spread when it appeared to help protect people against a typhoid fever epidemic. Brother Périn's pharmacy business grew. In 1788 he sold 5,638 florins' worth of medicine to outsiders and gave 506 florins of medicine to the poor. This income from medicines undoubtedly helped monastic orders flourish.

Cistercians and Franciscans were notable for their interest in herbal healing and gardening. The Abbey of Walkenreid, founded in 1127 in Saxony, a region within the former East Germany which had been swamp lands in the Thuringian basin, was converted by monks into the lush, fertile Golden Meadows that were divided into about eleven granges. Some plants needed for medicinal use did not grow in that area, so many were introduced from southern and tropical climates to this northern one. A few of the plants were hardy enough and grew wild. One such transplant, called plague root, was commonly used for patients during epidemics.

Most infirmaries within monasteries were located near the physic garden. It was believed that the beauty and scent of the garden helped soothe patients while they were treated with various herbal concoctions. It was here that *simples*, the term for single healing herbs made into medicinal brews, were prepared for the sick according to ancient directions. Many healing elixirs managed to survive the centuries.

What were some of the plants grown in these physic gardens? They were many, including horehound, lovage, mint, radish, garlic, chicory, parsley, and rose. Many white blossoms were deemed holy and especially revered.

Hop vines, believed to cool sexual ardor, were said to have flourished within the walled paths of fragrant gardens. One might suppose that monks who had taken the vow of chastity considered this herb a necessity. Although consumption of pepper in most parts of Europe during the Middle Ages was modest, monastic records indicate it was used medicinally in great quantities. Many other herbs were given to the ill at that time. Herbal tonics were turned into an art form by another, this time American, religious order.

## "HANDS TO WORK, HEARTS TO GOD" AND SUCCESS WITH HERBS

A small band of eight loyal believers followed Mother Ann Lee (1736–1784) to America, where they founded the largest, most successful group to manufacture and sell herbal products and medicines. The Shakers, originally known as the Society of Followers (or the Shaking Quakers) had beliefs similar to those of monastic orders. They preferred to live in communities separate from the world, and they held strict moral beliefs, including that of celibacy (a prohibition against marriage). While men and women were kept separate, they held equal rights and responsibilities within the communities. They spent their lives in work, worship, peace, humility, order, and brotherhood. Their belief that good work is a form of worship and a way to Christian perfection led them to become successful in many enterprises, including the making and selling of medicinal herbs. Their motto "hands to work, hearts to God" was practiced in everyday life.

The first Shaker settlement was in the wilderness at Watervliet, New York, near Albany. Eventually, 17 more communities and 51 families were created. Membership grew to 6,000 by 1850. Each society was expertly organized. All had similar functions, dress, and customs although each community served as an independent economic unit, drawing on the talents and various occupations of members that allowed them to sell surplus crafts.

Their main concern was in crafting only useful things. Ornament was considered unnecessary in the furniture and tools they crafted. And most Shaker communes were at first agricultural and horticultural. In praise of farming, their favored occupation, one Shaker wrote, "If you would have a lovely garden, you should live a lovely life." They enjoyed working the land and did so with great skill. Items sold included fruits, fruit butters, jams, applesauce, dried corn, wine, maple syrup, cucumber pickles, and catsup. Later they created baskets, knitwear, chairs, and many other pieces of useful furniture. They also invented time-saving tools for farming and were competent blacksmiths and leather tanners.

The difference between the Shakers and the many short-lived communistic groups in the United States was in their ability to organize completely and to use their abilities to advantage. The members at New Lebanon, New York (and later in communities in Ohio, Massachusetts, Connecticut, New Hampshire, Maine, Kentucky, Indiana, and Florida), were the first to realize the obvious possibilities of gardening and how it could bring the income necessary to keeping the community running well. Since they chose to do and make only useful things, naturally only useful plants were favored. The Shakers' love of gardening led to creation of a successful seed business. The next step seemed obvious, a medicinal herb business.

Thomas Corbett from the East Canterbury, New Hampshire, village took up study of medicinal herbs around 1813. With the help of a physician, he worked out the formula for Corbett's Compound Concentrated Syrup of Sarsaparilla, winning a medal at the Philadelphia Centennial in 1876. This compound, the most famous extract, some have considered to have been an impetus to the invention of the soft-drink industry.

Early Shaker ledgers show no record of the sale of herbs or extracts until 1821. Herbs, of course, were gathered earlier, but very few had been sold as packaged medicines by the Shakers before that time. Shaker Nathan Slosson delivered rosewater to Albany, New York, and other centers as early as 1809 for 50¢ a bottle. Similar items were produced and sold. A catalog of medicinal plants issued by the New Lebanon society claimed that they were the "first in this country to introduce . . . herbs and vegetable extracts for medicinal purposes placed on the market . . ." A note advised, "Orders for simples should be forwarded as early in the season as July."

The herb industry rapidly grew from 1844 to 1848. Rosewater had always been a popular item, but in the late 1840s the extract or tonic business began to take off. Member Shakers took great pains to ensure that their products were always of the highest quality. They carefully gathered and dried herbs for the elixirs they manufactured. In 1850 the New Lebanon community added a steam boiler, globe-shaped copper vacuum pan for drying herbs, and three double presses capable of pressing 100 pounds of herbs per day. The extract business outperformed other Shaker enterprises, and their physic garden grew to more than 50 acres. In 1850, they made 7,000 pounds of extracts.

Stimulated by better organization of work space and improved equipment, their extract business continued to expand. In the period 1861–1862, the Shakers manufactured a hundred different varieties of solid and liquid extracts. They usually sold the extracts in one- or five-pound bottles, although records also indicate eighth-, quarter-, and half-pound sizes and some ounce quantities were available. In 1861, 5,544 gallons of fluid extract were produced. The extracts were so successful that in 1870 the sisters made more than a million labels for extract bottles.

In the Shakers' early years, wild herbs were the main source. Many people believed that wild herbs were more powerful than cultivated varieties. While the Shakers cultivated most of their own herbs and roots, when business grew they began in 1826 to buy some herbs from outside sources. Within ten years, they began buying herbs from around the world, producing many simple extracts from herbs like hop, henbane, boneset (thoroughwort), lobelia, pennyroyal, spearmint, peppermint, catnip, wintergreen, sage, belladonna, marigold, chamomile, yellow dock, and garden lettuce. Various roots, like burdock, bloodroot, parsley, dandelion, and yarrow, were also made into medicinal elixirs. Records also mention compound syrups of sarsaparilla, black cohosh, rosewater, the superfine flower of slippery elm, and peach water.

Some famous Shaker tonics, besides Corbett's Compound Concentrated Syrup of Sarsaparilla, were Mother Seigel's Curative Syrup (extract of roots), Norwood's Tincture of Veratrum (a tincture of hellebore used to treat pneumonia, heart and circulatory problems, typhoid fever, rheumatism, measles, yellow fever, and other diseases), and Seven Barks (blue flag, butternut, goldenseal, sassafras, lady's slipper, bloodroot, black cohosh, and mandrake), manufactured for Dr. Lyman Brown and said to promote long life. This last tonic, widely sold in the United States and Canada, was exported to England, France, and Germany. Another tonic, the Shaker Asthma Cure, also sold well as advertisements claimed "No disease is harder to cure." Labels on Shaker medicines were always plainly printed with ingredients and informative, easy-to-follow directions.

By the 1890s the Shakers' income from extracts was still considerable. In 1899 a new boiler was installed at the extract laboratory. And the Shakers had earned a reputation for honesty and reliability as well as a high-quality product. People continued to demand tonics and medicines. Their success and popularity, however, encouraged counterfeiters, who wanted to profit on Shaker look-alikes that they created, which were of questionable quality.

On the whole, the Shakers were a healthy, hard-working people who worked outdoors and lived in sanitary conditions. Their simple, stress-free life, eating of fresh, homegrown foods, and use of herbal tonics allowed most members to live very long lives. Due to their strict moral codes, many communities were unable to recruit new members. Slowly, the sect dwindled. Gradually, they hired outside laborers and eventually closed villages. However, the spirit of Shakerism survives and some new interest has been kindled.

## TONIC DOWNFALL

In the mid-19th century medicine experienced a major change. Herbal and folk medicines slowly evolved into a business, thanks to the Shakers. As the U.S. Civil War raged on, demand for medical supplies, health practitioners, and medicines increased. But success breeds many imitators looking for riches. Those unable to create herbal blends formulated "tonics" that resembled them. Some created medicines that produced an immediate physical response so that they could convince potential patients to make repeat purchases. At this time, cocaine was cheap, plentiful, and legal. Alcohol, which could be produced very cheaply, also produced euphoric results almost immediately. Both substances became basic ingredients in many bogus patent medicines or tonics produced during this era.

Today's soft drinks were originally linked with tonics. Drinks like root beer, sarsaparilla, and sassafras were created from an array of herbs reported to boost health. Mixed with soda water, they were served at pharmacies, advertised as "pick-me-ups." Coca-Cola, formulated by Atlanta pharmacist John Pemberton, originally included traces of cocaine. Coca-Cola was first advertised as a "brain tonic and intellectual beverage which could also cure menstrual distress." In 1903 cocaine was replaced by a nonnarcotic extract of coca leaves, but an entire generation grew up on this so-called tonic beverage. And we continue to imbibe such drinks, which we sometimes convince ourselves are tonics, today.

The Shakers fought valiantly against the many fakes and tried to make their products separate. In 1884 Shaker Benjamin Gates wrote to fellow Shakers that the company producing Smith Brothers cough drops had used the word *Shaker* as a trademark. Apparently, this matter was taken to court and resolved in favor of the Shakers, as recorded in later letters.

But many fakes endured. What better product could one package and sell than a bottle of bitters capable of curing all diseases? How easy it would be to carry such a bottle across vast plains and around mountains where no physician could be found. Many bitters began in small bottles, but as the amount of alcohol increased, the bottles got larger, too. And as the alcohol increased, medicinal values often dwindled. Many products did not contain the liquids they claimed on their labels.

Fake medicines were advertised far and wide with flyers and medicine shows. They were packaged in appealing containers with bright labels that announced miraculous cures and made wild claims. Many hucksters were quite skillful at pushing their products. "Indian medicines" were sold by American Indians in carnival settings with stage-show antics and war cries. An old chief sold something called Ka-ton-ka on street corners with a book that asked, "Whoever saw a bald Indian? Whoever saw an Indian with bad teeth? Whoever saw an Indian with a deranged liver?" Indians "just take good old Ka-ton-ka freely and live to be a hundred." Another tonic, Vegetine, claimed to be a great blood-purifier, was recommended for all skin diseases and almost everything else. Sarsaparilla extracts became big business. An unscrupulous group of men had a physician sell them his name for $7 a week so that they could place it on their label. That's how Dr. Townsend's Compound Extract of Sarsaparilla began. This extract, advertised as the "wonder and blessing of the age, the most extraordinary medicine in the world," made the producers a fortune.

As the Indian medicine rage dwindled, other gimmicks caught on, among them products supposedly formulated by "Quaker doctors." So, religion became a marketing tool intended to instill confidence. Songs and snappy phrases abounded as tonic producers fought for a market share. A long list of bitters was created and marketed. Over 130 brands were produced in the United States and Canada, including Iron Tonic Bitters, German Herb Bitters, Stoughton Bitters, Wild Cherry Bitters, and Hop Tonic Bitters.

We cannot claim that all tonics not made by Shakers were useless, however. A few honest people also marketed their herbal medicines. Lydia E. Pinkham of Massachusetts was called a master of teakettle medicine and grandmother of modern advertising. She married in 1843 and reared children while working a little as a nurse. Having found an herbal recipe her husband received in settlement of an old debt, with her family facing hunger, Pinkham decided to go into business making and selling the herbal extract. In 1875, it arrived on the market as Lydia E. Pinkham's Vegetable Compound and was advertised as a remedy for "all female weakness." Her children filled bottles and folded circulars while she stirred up batch after batch in her kitchen. The compound enjoyed great success and is still sold today. So, if something works, it may indeed survive, though perhaps in a quiet way.

As better-quality ingredients were left out of the brew, tonics began to acquire a bad name. It was discovered that some were addictive, and many did not cure anything. No one knew which brand to trust; so they trusted none. Herbal tonics eventually became synonymous with the term *snake oil*, and a snake-oil peddler was someone not to be trusted.

In 1906, the U.S. Pure Food and Drug Law and the prosecution of bogus tonic manufacturers brought the herbal tonic business in the United States to an awful end. Although it began with high ideals and good results, it suffered a terrible blow from greedy hucksters. These hucksters effectively toyed with people's pain and suffering and laughed in their faces. They also destroyed faith in herbal healing, which only now is beginning to experience a revival. But how many people have suffered needlessly because of their greed?

For a brief time, during Prohibition, tonic wine bitters returned to kitchen pantries in the United States. But the bitter wines and medicinals were produced as a way of legally marketing alcohol under the guise of medicine. This ruse did not aid the cause of herbal tonics. Perhaps we can only be grateful that tonics and their genuine healing powers have not been lost forever.

In Canada, England, Europe, Australia, and New Zealand herbal tonics and alterative herbs fared somewhat better in the 20th century and were generally more accepted even by some orthodox medical practitioners. Nevertheless, they too have undergone a revival in interest as scientists document the positive effects of herbs and their essential oils. And more double-blind studies of chemicals within herbs if not of the whole herbs themselves have drawn more enthusiastic acceptance from the Western medical community.

# Our Bodies, Our Herbs
## How Herbs Help and Heal

If we use real tonics, brews which contain good-quality herbs and ingredients, we know we'll get results. Somehow physical changes occur. We begin to feel better and to recover from illnesses. How do these herbs work?

This isn't a mysterious process. The herbs merely contain phytochemicals, known as essential oils, which help the body heal itself. The precious liquids inside healing herbs vary in composition and often have a wide range of medicinal uses. Some herbs boost the immune system, others inhibit tumor growth and metastases, and still others cleanse the lymphatic system. These essential oils have been found in labs to contain terpenes, phenols, alcohols, and aldehydes. Many of these substances are antiseptic and make good bactericides.

But essential oils are complex compounds that often have a dominant chemical that endows the herb with its primary therapeutic use. What's important is that the whole plant (the sum of all its chemicals) seems responsible for its healing effects. The delicate balance of chemicals—one chemical helps a second work, a third ensures that that effect is not too strong, and a fourth does something else—creates natural, soothing healing. Nature in the plant and its essential oil has created something complete that allows you to direct it toward healing for a particular purpose. In contrast, many pharmaceutical companies review uses only of isolated chemicals and how they affect the body. Consider the Chinese ephedra plant (*Ephedra major*), an old, primitive species related to the horsetail and known for decongestant abilities for over 5,000 years. Modern researchers isolated a single substance contained within the plant, ephedrine, which acts as a nerve stimulant similar to adrenaline, and they've used this lone chemical or its synthetic equivalent to create many decongestant medicines. Herbalists, however, have found that using the whole plant medicinally produces fewer heart problems. The whole plant or the essential oil is also more effective and gentler than the isolated chemical. The whole plant stimulates, energizes, and increases vitality. The isolated chemical, ephedrine, on the other hand, tends to make one feel jittery, and it has other side effects.

This is true with almost all plants. They contain a wide variety of chemical compounds which interact in various ways. Let's look at the main chemical compounds and what they do. *Alcohols* provide effective germicidal action. *Aldehydes* are antiinflammatory and disinfectant and act as buffers to control the acidity of the plant's natural acids. *Esters* are helpful in controlling fungus and yeast within the body, *lactones* and *hydrocarbons* are antiinflammatory, and *phenols* have disinfectant and antiseptic actions. Nearly all these chemical compounds occur in various combinations within the essential oils of plants.

These compounds are so complex that we probably do not even understand how they all work together and what these various actions do within the plants themselves. But we do know through modern research how powerful they are. The essence of eucalyptus, which has antiseptic properties, has been demonstrated to be much more powerful in its whole form. The principal chemical, eucalyptol, when isolated and used by itself is simply not as effective. This appears to be true of virtually all herbs used in herbal medicine. Plant chemicals act synergistically, and the whole is greater than the sum of its parts. The individual chemicals apparently help each other. Nature has a way of balancing varied chemical compositions for individual plant needs. It's been said that if we were to discover the secrets contained within all varied forms of plant life and their essential oils, it would take over a thousand years.

Perhaps that would be time well spent. In contemporary life our bodies deal with many toxins that tax the immune system, which defends the body against disease. Industrial chemicals and other contaminants, pollution, overuse of antibiotics, other drugs found in our food and daily lives, birth control pills, and stress make the use of herbs and tonics especially well suited to enhancing our general well-being.

In a recent survey in *Medical Herbalism: A Clinical Newsletter for the Herbal Practitioner*, readers were asked to rank the ten herbs thought most important in their practice. Of 89 respondents, 74 listed echinacea as the most commonly used as a tonic and immune-system stimulant. Other frequently cited tonics were goldenseal (antibiotic, astringent), dandelion (alterative), nettle (alterative, astringent), ginseng (energizer), hawthorn (good for heart), garlic (antibiotic), valerian (sedative, analgesic), milk thistle (good for liver), and licorice (energizer, good for respiratory and digestive systems).

Herbal tonics are important for healing because they contain powerful herbs that stimulate the body to heal itself throughout. We're not certain how herbs do this, but they restore the body's balance, facilitate excretion of toxic wastes, purify blood and fluids, and tone up the organs. Because we don't quite understand these actions and because the actions are nonspecific, mainstream medical science has failed to accept many of these herbal tonics. As more people use and get results from these tonics, it becomes harder to ignore them. Generally, tonics act over a long period to change things within the body, restoring, renewing, and cleansing.

# CLEANSING

Herbal tonics don't cure us, they merely assist the body in naturally restoring itself. We can assist this process and increase the body's effectiveness while we are on a tonic program.

What we're doing, in effect, is cleansing the body, whether we're fighting a specific illness or simply using a tonic or tonics once or twice a year to help us feel healthier and more energetic. *Cleansing* is an apt term. Most of us bathe every day, washing away the impurities and dirt that collect over a 24-hour period. Internally, we can collect toxins when we do not eliminate wastes properly. "Constipation is often referred to as the 'modern plague.' Indeed, it is the greatest present-day danger to health. Intestinal toxemia and the resulting autotoxication is a direct result . . . ," Dr. Bernard Jensen states in *Tissue Cleansing through Bowel Management* (1981).

When the body is unable to dispose of wastes which contain toxins, this lowers immune-system functioning because it is overloaded. This in turn can affect all organs, like the lungs, liver, kidneys, and skin, as well as the lymphatic system, which help in natural cleansing. Dr. Jensen adds that the underlying cause of this inability is poor nutrition. Drinking enough water and getting enough exercise are also contributing factors.

Herbal tonics, packed with nutrition undisturbed by pesticides and chemical processing, are the answer. While taking these tonics, we can help the body eliminate toxins and speed up healing effects. The more serious the illness, the more important it is to follow a tonic regimen. I think the four most important steps—fasting, aromatic baths, extra rest along with physical exercise, and lots of pure fluids—are needed to restore good health. Later, we'll consider two methods of using herbs within a tonic program.

## PLENTY OF PURE FLUIDS

All people, especially those who want to lose weight, should drink eight glasses of water a day. That's a standard health dictum. But I have known people who never drink water. Instead, they gulp down sugary sodas, coffee by the gallon, and drinks containing sugar substitutes, but they turn their noses up at the thought of downing a single glass of pure, sparkling water. Don't get me wrong; I am one of the worst offenders. Somehow through the years I, too, became addicted to diet sodas. As my addiction reached its peak, I found myself rarely drinking water and reaching for a diet soda instead when I was thirsty. Fortunately, my husband (who has many bad health habits but takes his water seriously) has reminded me to drink water when I'm off track. Unhappily, many of us are dehydrated because we don't drink enough water.

Physicians agree that the way to keep the kidneys and liver healthy as well as to keep the skin clear is to drink plenty of water. This also helps the colon. After all, the body is made up mostly of fluids, and water is one of the best ways to force out waste. So, it is recommended that, in addition to your tonic, you drink eight glasses of water per day. Avoid sugary drinks, those containing caffeine, and diet drinks.

## REST AND EXERCISE

Exercise is vital to health, but so is rest. The key to many good health habits is balance. Walking is a gentle and easy way to get started. Monitor your pace and as you become accustomed to your routine, a brisk walk will help condition your heart and lungs. Make it fun, give yourself goals, and enjoy the feeling of well-being. My favorite exercise is yoga, since it involves a gentle stretching program. I've found books and videos for learning the postures. I find it a great way to condition the body without taxing it. I'm not one for sweating and puffing and dancing around; so, many other exercise programs don't appeal to me. The movements in yoga are graceful and beautiful and make the body feel very good. Many yoga postures work well for the aged or physically challenged, too. Discuss an exercise program appropriate for you with your physician.

The body also needs rest. When on a tonic program, go to bed early and get up early to ensure that you get maximum benefits. You may also want to explore relaxation techniques and meditation, since they can help you manage daily stress.

## FASTING

Fasting involves going without food for a certain period of time. Short fasts can help restore health and rejuvenate the body. Fasting can be a natural way of life, even though we've been told otherwise. Watch animals. When they do not feel well, they often stop eating. Fasting is one of the oldest therapies known to humans, and it can help anyone who needs to renew. Hippocrates and Paracelsus often prescribed fasting as a way of healing. Recent studies have suggested that periodic fasting helped increase the life span of animals.

To fast you don't have to do without food completely. The best way to fast, that's easy on the body and good for a tonic program, is a liquid fast consisting of pure fruit juices, vegetable juices, and broths. Short fasts can be easy and safe to accomplish, provided that you don't have diabetes, a problem with low blood sugar, or other serious diseases. Longer fasts, up to 30 days, can also be undertaken. First check with your physician and read several books on fasting, like *How to Keep Slim, Healthy & Young with Juice Fasting* (1984) by Dr. Paavo Airola.

# AROMATIC BATHS

As you work to get the toxins out, you will experience certain changes. You may suddenly have bad breath, you'll need to go to the bathroom more often, and you may perspire more heavily with stronger odors as the toxins leach out. Chewing parsley or drinking parsley tea will help the breath, but you need to cleanse the skin of toxins that leave the body through pores and perspiration. This is where aromatic baths can help. I recommend adding 6 to 15 drops of pure essential oil to a tub of warm water each evening and soaking for 10 to 15 minutes. Susanne Fischer-Rizzi in *Complete Aromatherapy Handbook* (Sterling, 1990) recommends adding sea salt along with essential oils to bathwater to cleanse and remove toxins. She also claims that the minerals in sea salt strengthen the immune system. Salt is a great cleanser that helps deodorize; so, grab a handful and toss it in the water. Then add the essential oil and swish the water around to dissolve the salt.

If you have dry or sensitive skin, you may want to try oatmeal. Place a handful of oatmeal in a washcloth and knot it well. After you tie it up, allow it to float in the tub, making the water milky. Then you can dispose of the oatmeal after your bath without clogging the drain.

You can use many different essential oils, assuming you're not allergic and the oil is not abrasive. Here are four good choices: geranium (balances the body, relieves tension, and lifts the mood), lavender (heals, calms, and tones muscles), lemon (cools, cleanses, and is refreshing), and rose (calms, balances, and is good for the skin). What an enjoyable way to cleanse!

# TONIC PROGRAMS

Here are two methods you can use for a tonic program. The first, a short program, can refresh and renew you any time you feel the need, whether it's once a year or once a month. I call this the weekend renewal program. It's easy to incorporate into a busy life although it is very effective in keeping the body balanced and healthy. The second method, the wellness tonic program, takes longer and can best be used when the body needs help in fighting disease.

### Weekend Renewal Program
The weekend renewal program is a two- to three-day herbal tonic program that can refresh and invigorate the body. First choose the tonic herb or herbs you need for your body. Read the following chapters on herbs to

decide whether you'll want to use a simple tonic containing one particular herb or a tonic tincture composed of several herbs. Also study the herbs' healing attributes, directions for preparation, and recommended dosages.

Then set aside two or three days that will be fairly stress free. Try to delegate your responsibilities or set them aside for these days. Since most people have full days, this program will require your making a time commitment.

Plan your meals and write out a menu plan. To help you remember to drink your 8 glasses of water, measure your water for the day, and place it in a container in the refrigerator. At the end of the day, the container should need to be refilled. Lemon or lime slices can add zing and visual appeal to an occasional glass of water. Meals should consist of fresh fruit juices for breakfast, vegetable juices for lunch, and clear broths and soups for dinner. Herbal tonics can be taken a half-hour before meals and before bedtime, as indicated.

Exercise for 1 hour each day, whatever else you choose to do. Add time for meditation or quiet, and try to take an afternoon nap of no more than an hour. Take a break from television, and find things to keep you pleasantly busy. Do some gardening, read, work on hobbies, do puzzles, or watch a funny movie, if those things please you. I find television too much stimulation and it seems to entice people to eat all the wrong foods. At the end of the day, take a relaxing bath and snuggle in for a good night's sleep.

### Wellness Tonic Program

The wellness tonic program requires a greater time commitment, but regaining health makes it worth the time. You also have to organize and plan ahead. Choose a healing tonic carefully because you're struggling to get well from a disease. The blended herbal brew must meet your specific needs. Take time to obtain top-quality ingredients.

Using a notebook, map out the days for your tonic program. You can follow the basics of the weekend renewal program, but adapt it to your needs. You may require more or longer rest periods, or you may be unable to be as physically active. If so, plan for necessary naps or add shorter, less taxing periods of physical movement. You know what you can do. I believe meditation is important daily; it also seems to help the body deal with stress. You may also want to keep a journal to record your thoughts and feelings. Remember that you may experience a healing crisis: you'll actually feel worse as your body begins to cleanse itself of toxins. This is normal and to be expected. Your journal can be a revealing diary, and it may even help you come to terms with how you got sick.

If you want to follow a long-term fast, do your research, invest in a good juicer, and talk with your physician. Serious fasters have advised enemas for cleansing the body of built-up toxins. You may want to try this if you're still not eliminating daily. An evening enema will help rid the body of accumulated wastes, but some people even take two enemas, one in the morning and one at night. Find a colonic specialist to do the job, or you can do it yourself at home with an enema bag, available at most drugstores.

If you don't want to fast, make sure the foods you do eat are organic, fresh, and light. Try to stay away from meat, oily and fried foods, sweets, and caffeine. Include many fruits and vegetables, and remember to drink water.

## HERBALISTS' CASE STUDIES

It's amazing that good health can be just a tonic away. That's why I wanted to relate a few stories herbalists have shared with me during interviews. Many herbalists recounted that the simplicity of the cure astounded their patients. Nearly all discovered in the end that healing comes naturally. All names have been changed to protect privacy.

Martha, a 56-year-old woman, suffered for years with crippling arthritis. Her hands were knotted and it was difficult for her to walk or even simply move. Her days were centered around her disease: would it be a *good* day with less pain or a *bad* day spent in bed in agony? After trying conventional treatments which merely tried to mask the pain and didn't even accomplish that, she decided to try the herbal route. A friend referred her to an herbalist, who in turn put her on cleansing tonics. The herbalist also recommended apple pectin and a 3-day fast. Martha followed her advice and "suddenly" within weeks after years of pain, she found herself pain free. With tears in her eyes she told the herbalist the tonics had given her back her life.

Ovarian cancer is a deadly and devastating disease. Annie, 42, was diagnosed with it 4 years ago. The word *cancer* sent chills down her spine, since she had watched many family members battle the disease in various forms and lose. She vowed to win this battle. She followed conventional therapies, and at the same time she also took daily doses of Essiac Tonic, a cancer remedy that an herbalist friend prescribed for her. She credits the tonic for her continued good health. During her chemotherapy she did not experience the normal side effects like nausea or hair loss and was able to return to work quickly. Four years later she continues to take the tonic periodically.

Thomas, 48, was diagnosed by his physician as having adult-onset diabetes. After a lifetime of good health, suddenly it seemed as if he was falling apart. He was experiencing skin rashes, digestive upsets, and many other symptoms. He felt there was a better way to treat himself, so, he went to an herbalist who put him on a five-herb tonic which also contained sodium sulfate. Within weeks, he felt renewed. He made an appointment to see the doctor, who retested him and told him he didn't have diabetes and that there must have been a mistake. The herbalist knew there wasn't a mistake. The herbal tonic had been reported to defeat adult-onset diabetes with a 100 percent cure rate. That particular herbalist had just started using it, but found it successful.

An 80-year-old woman who suffered with shingles that affected her right leg for several years, fasted for three days while taking the same formula and found almost instant relief.

Claudia, a young woman in her early thirties, was diagnosed with chronic fatigue syndrome. This debilitating illness makes life impossible for sufferers, who struggle to fight the overwhelming fatigue that makes the simplest everyday tasks major obstacles. A medical doctor and an osteopath did not help. After taking an immune-boosting tonic for 6 months, her symptoms disappeared and she again led a normal life.

John, age 15, suffered from an extreme case of acne. His face was a raw mass of eruptions. Not only painful, it was most embarrassing, especially at his young age. The creams his dermatologist prescribed just weren't working well enough. His mother took him to see an herbalist, who put him on a cleansing tonic. His face lost the angry red welts and was soon clear. He could now do all the things a normal teenage boy does, without worrying about how his face would look. No scars were left behind.

These are merely a small sample of the many healing stories I've heard. To list all such stories would take volumes. So, let's get on to the business of learning about how to make and use healing tonics for ourselves.

# How-To's of Tonic Preparation

When you begin to work with healing herbs, you get a sense of what natural healing in the body is really all about. There isn't some magic in the herb itself. The basis is super nutrition. Every plant contains individual attributes and abilities. Certain chemicals, along with the vitamins and minerals in the herbs, when concentrated within a tonic, aid the body in becoming strong enough to fight off disease. The tonic does this by helping the body rid itself of pesty invading organisms or by preventing illness entirely. Some of these herbal properties are very healing and highly nutritious for humans.

Other herbs and tonics are stronger and potentially dangerous if not used carefully. Also, some plants are deadly or poisonous. We have to be responsible and we need to respect the plant world. We can learn a lot from it. While we do not want to live in fear, we do want to arm ourselves with knowledge. That's why, when you begin to explore this green world, you should do what ancient shamans advised new apprentices: become aware.

Read all you can about herbs and plants. Familiarize yourself with the plants you are most interested in. Start with plants you need right now. In the chapters that follow, locate tonic herbs that would be most helpful to your situation. Begin by knowing these plants and what their leaves, flowers, berries, fruit, roots, and seeds look like. What do they smell like? How do the leaves feel? What is the plant's growing habits? As you become aware of the many physical attributes of the plant, you may begin to get a feeling for the essence of the plant itself. This is the plant's own life force, and this method has been used by many native tribes in the Americas who used plants for healing. This way, you may be able to tap into your natural or instinctual communication with the plant, as it were. Animals still use this method, since they seem to instinctively know which plants to eat when ill. Although humans seem to have lost this instinct, I'd like to think we can recultivate it if we work at it.

Since we still have the benefit of much research from past generations, along with modern science, we can begin our healing journey right away. Perhaps we can work on this link with nature as we work with herbs. Basically, by using tonics you become super nourished. You'll be able to create the concentrated nutritious drinks your body has been craving, perhaps even starving for. And this won't be hard to do once you've learned the basics.

# HERBAL EXTRACTS

Both medicinal and nutritious properties can be extracted from plants in many ways. Here we'll consider several and choose those most suited to our needs. All methods are intended to separate the juice from the plant so that you'll be able to use it in concentrated form.

## Water Method

This method, called *infusion*, is perhaps the most common and popular home method of preparing herbs for our use. Often it is used to prepare herbal teas. Infusion involves pouring boiling water over the herb (covering it to prevent the essential oils from escaping in the steam) and letting it steep for a short time, usually 15 to 20 minutes for medicinal applications. The herbs used in this method are ones most receptive to releasing their essential oils, usually leaves and flowers whether fresh or dried. However, some barks and roots can also be steeped, as long as they are powdered. Then strain the tea and discard the plant material.

Another water method is used for tougher plant material, like tough twigs, roots, barks, and seeds. The chemicals locked within usually require more than just pouring boiling water over them. For these materials, you'll need to place them in a pan of water and bring the mixture to a boil. Then cover it and reduce heat to simmer, generally about 30 minutes. Then strain the water. This produces a strong, dark-colored tea.

These liquids are meant to be used immediately or within 3 to 7 days if refrigerated. They do not contain any preservatives. You can triple the amount of herb used to make your infusion and then add honey (equal amounts of honey to the liquid) to create a concentrated syrup. Then add the syrup to 1 cup of warm water (about 2 tablespoons per cup). It's easy and already sweetened. The syrup will last longer than the plain infusion, but it should still be refrigerated.

## Tincture Method

*Tinctures* are made by steeping the plant material in alcohol or apple cider vinegar. What you come up with is very concentrated material preserved for long periods of time. Add 30 drops to 1 cup of warm water or juice to make an instant tea tonic. The alcohol and vinegar base are two solutions which help break the plant down, making it easy to extract the valuable essential oils contained within.

Detailed instructions for making the alcohol tincture is in the last chapter. This method is best when using a multiherb blend, but you can also use the same method for simply one particular herb.

Vinegar tinctures are pretty much the same as alcohol tinctures; you simply exchange the alcohol for vinegar and use the same dosage in a cup of warm water. There are several reasons you might want to use a vinegar tincture. Apple cider vinegar is healing in itself. It contains potassium and other minerals; it is also antiseptic and cleansing. Also, many people do not wish to take alcohol in any form, for religious or other reasons.

When using apple cider vinegar, make sure you are using vinegar made from whole, crushed apples. The label should tell you. That way you'll get more health benefits from the apple. Here's an easy way to make your own if you have a do-it-yourself spirit or want to monitor quality. Take some organically grown, freshly washed apples and crush them slightly, skins and all. Place them in a clean crock and cover with water. Add extra apple peelings if you wish, then cover with muslin or a lid. Place the crock in a warm, out-of-the-way place; it should stay at about 70 degrees. Every 2 to 3 days, skim off the foam that accumulates at the top. After about 5 weeks this liquid will smell and taste like vinegar. That's when you know it is done. Strain it two to three times. Then pour the cider vinegar into bottles and seal them to use whenever you need. Cork or plastic lids are best since vinegar tends to rust metal.

## TOOLS OF THE TRADE

Preparing a tonic requires a method of cooking, and like any other kitchen project, it requires certain tools to make the job easier. Here's a list of things you may want to buy when making infusions. You can do without these tools and utensils, but it's nicer to have them.

### Teapot

The best teapots are made of enamel, china, earthenware, or glass. Make sure the teapot has no chips or cracks. When making tonics, the brew is steeped a long time; so, it's helpful to have a tea cosy. This is simply a cotton cover which goes over the teapot to help keep the tea warm for a longer period. Tea cosys can be easily made or bought. Some teapots have strainers built in over the spout. Whatever you do, never heat the teapot directly. Teapots are meant only for steeping (pouring the boiling water into the pot with herbs and letting it sit for a specified time) and for serving.

### Infuser or Strainer

An infuser contains the plant material so that it doesn't end up in your teacup. It also saves you from having to strain it too. Infusers come in all shapes and sizes. I have seen some shaped like a spoon (a handle with a ball at the end) or even like tiny teapots themselves, but they're mostly ball-shaped and come with tiny holes all over the surface. The infuser screws or snaps apart so that you can fill it with herb material and then close it tight to prevent bits from escaping (but the essential oils do). Sizes range from small infusers suitable for 1 to 2 cups of tea to the infuser meant for large pots, holding enough herb for 6 to 8 cups of tea. You can also purchase empty teabags which you can fill yourself and seal with a hot iron. However, I don't like these since they never hold enough for tonic use, and I've had trouble with the sealed ends coming loose and making the mess I was trying to avoid.

If you add the herbal material loosely to the teapot, you can also simply use a kitchen strainer to remove the plant material while pouring the tea into your cup.

### Mortar and Pestle or Grinder

A mortar and pestle is an old method used to grind small amounts of dried herbs and seeds. I like this tool for its old-time appeal and keep several on hand for small projects. You can purchase them where herb products are sold and in specialty mail-order catalogs. For dried roots and twigs that must be crushed, a good-quality food processor will reduce them to powder. Blenders can also be used to powder dried leaf herbs.

## EASING THE TASTE OF THE BITTERS

There's no way around it; most tonic herbs taste bitter. To improve the taste, without interfering with the healing attributes, here are some things you can do. Do not add sugar or milk since these ingredients are hard on the body and detract from the healing effects of the tea. Honey is a good sweetener to use. A few tonic herbs are pleasant-tasting and can be added for their pleasure value alone (but you'll get bonus healing effects, too). Peppermint, sassafras, and licorice root are good choices. Spices like cinnamon and clove may be added to your brew, as well as dried orange peels and lemon rinds. The tonic may never have a taste you'll like, but it can be made palatable. But your brew is drunk, not for pleasure, but for health. Any of these methods or a combination should help you accomplish your goal.

## GATHERING HERBS FOR TONICS

To obtain materials for herbal tonic preparation, there are three ways to do it: gather herbs from the wild, grow your own, or purchase dried plant material from a reputable source.

## Best Buys

If you purchase your material, try to get it in whole form. Leaves and seeds are easily bought this way. You can then crush the herbs yourself as you need them, and they will contain more precious essential oils. Roots will come in chunks, what's called cut form, although they're also available in powdered form. Since roots are often more powerful than the plant growing aboveground, buying root in powdered form should not cause a problem.

Store your dried material, whether in whole form or powdered, in labeled jars in a cool, dark place and make sure it has a tight-fitting lid. Also, it is absolutely necessary that the plant material be no more than a year old, especially when you're using it for medicinal purposes. This is why it's best to purchase dried herbs from well-known companies with high turnover. Don't be afraid to ask shopkeepers about the freshness of their product. It is, however, almost impossible to really tell how old the plant material is. The shopkeeper would not know how long the original wholesaler had it, only how long they had the herb in the store. The best way to check is to look at the product. Is it fresh-looking? By this I mean does it have good color, a strong scent, and good texture? If it is old, it will have lost most of its smell, be dark in color, and may have a lot of powder from having been around a long time.

## Foraging

Obviously, fresh is best whenever possible. You know the plant is still imbued with the life force. The problem with foraging from the wild is twofold. First, if you aren't sure of the herb, you can get into trouble with mistaken identities. Of course, you can always take classes on herbs, and get books from the bookstore or library on plant identification, and become familiar with the many different species. The subject is fascinating even if you aren't foraging wild. But today the areas for foraging are rapidly shrinking, and this means the chance of getting into trouble from trespassing increases. Unless you have a large amount of land with woods, foraging isn't the best choice. Many wild plants are endangered now, too, and I recommend that we avoid disturbing wild areas as much as possible.

## Your Own Backyard

This leaves one option if you want to go fresh, and that's to grow your own plots of medicinal plants. This method is best because you can order the exact species you need, in the quantity you want, and you'll observe the (continued on p. 49)

# COLORFUL HERBS

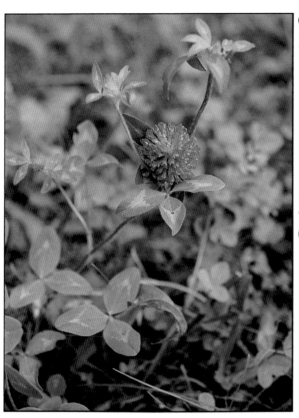

Red Clover
*Trifolium pratense*
(p. 109)

Apothecary Rose *Rosa gallica officinalis* (p. 92)

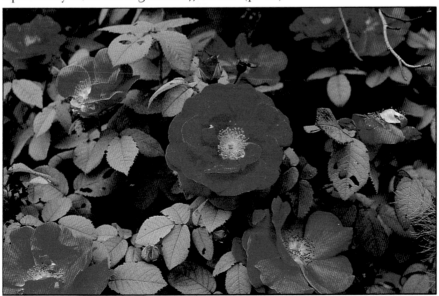

Lemon Balm
*Melissa officinalis*
(p. 114)

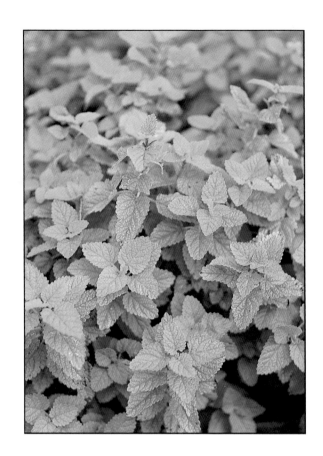

Lavender *Lavandula angustifolia* (p. 113)

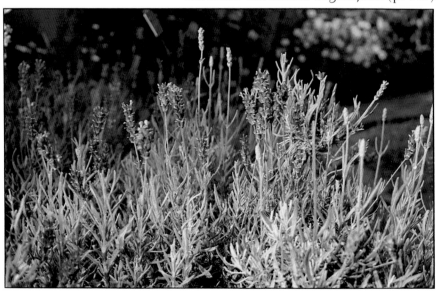

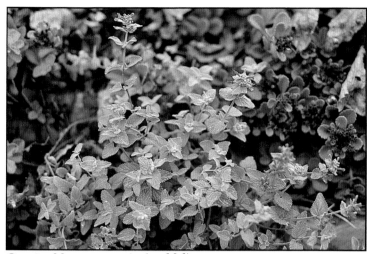

Catnip *Nepeta cataria* (p. 106)

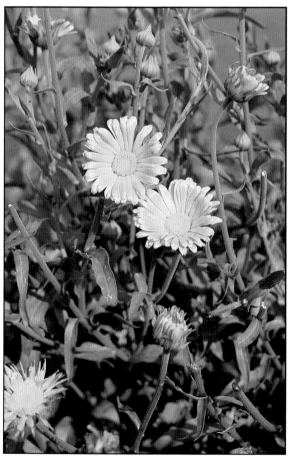

Calendula
*Calendula officinalis*
(p. 72)

Valerian
*Valeriana officinalis* (p. 117)

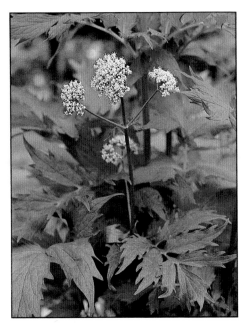

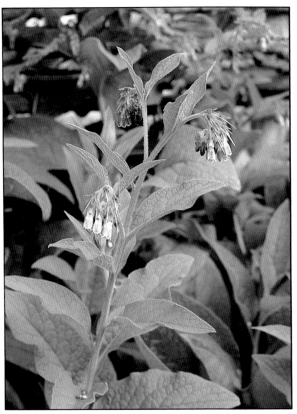

Comfrey
*Symphytum officinale* (p. 73

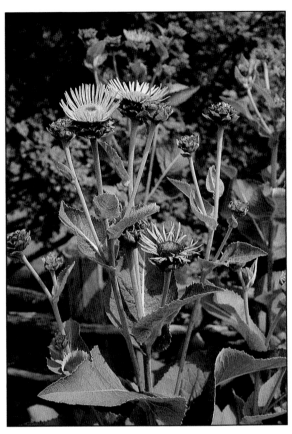

Elecampane
*Inula helenium* (p. 76)

Sweet Woodruff *Galium odoratum* (p. 69)

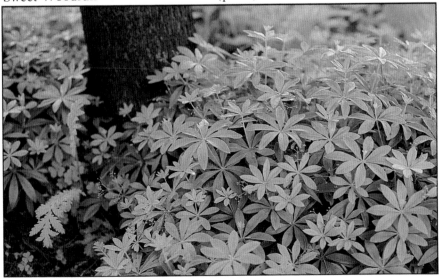

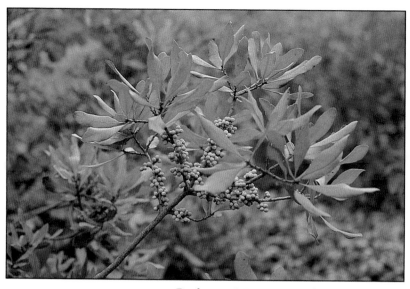

Bayberry *Myrica pensylvanica* (p. 120)

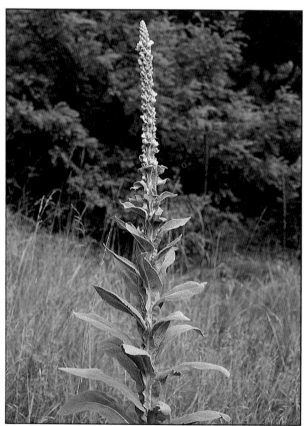

Mullein
*Verbascum thapsus*
(p. 80)

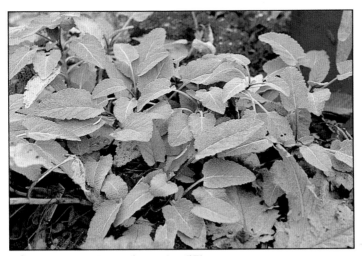

Clary Sage *Salvia sclarea* (p. 57)

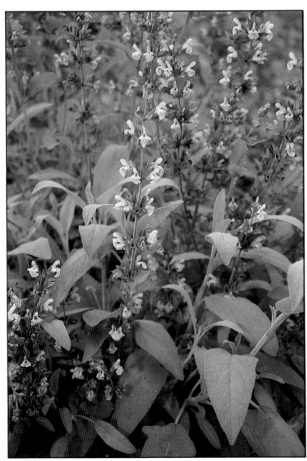

Sage
*Salvia officinalis*
(p. 128)

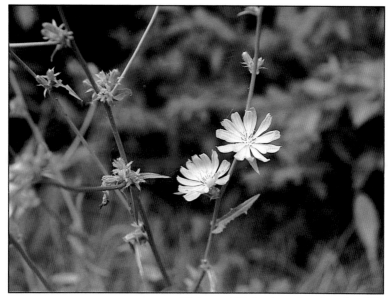

Chicory *Cichorium intybus* (p. 56)

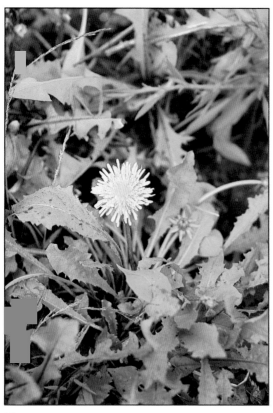

Dandelion
*Taraxacum officinale* (p. 61)

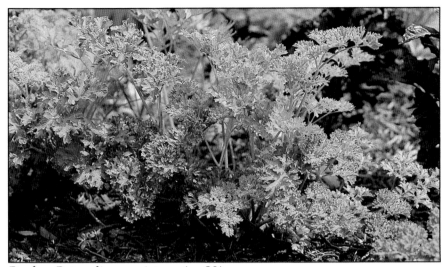

Parsley *Petroselinum crispum* (p. 90)

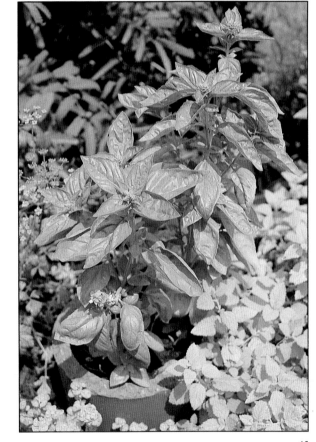

Sweet Basil
*Ocimum basilicum*
(p. 101)

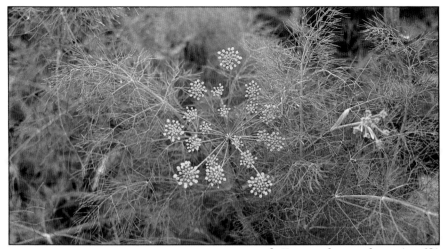

Fennel *Foeniculum vulgare* (p. 63)

Dill
*Anethum graveolens*
(p. 110)

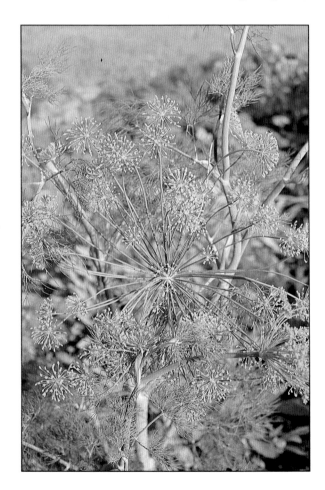

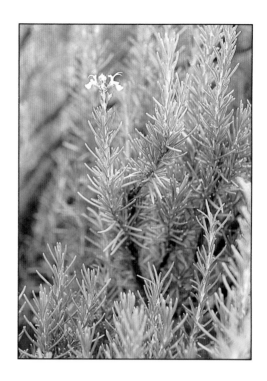

Rosemary
*Rosmarinus officinalis* (p. 127)

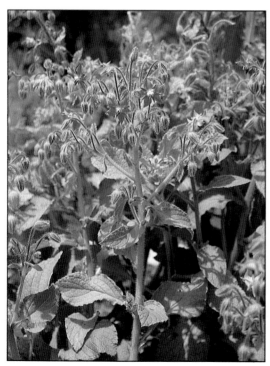

Borage
*Borago officinalis* (p. 105)

43

Peppermint
*Mentha piperita* (p. 89)

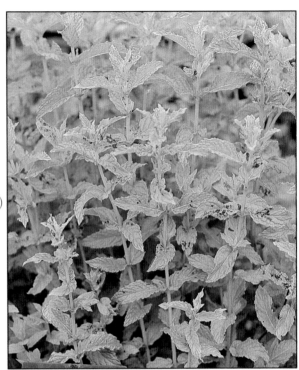

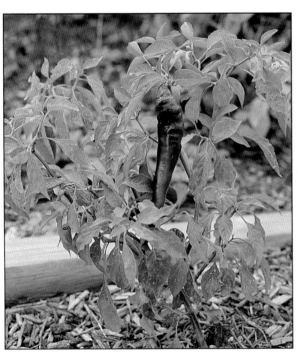

Cayenne Pepper
*Capsicum annuum*
(p. 84)

Rhubarb
*Rheum officinale* (p. 67)

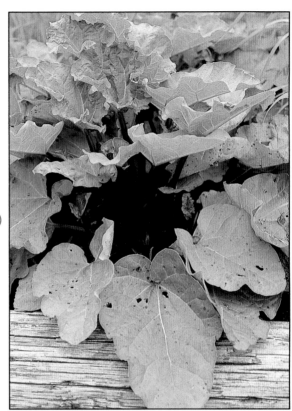

Apple *Malus pumila* (p. 53)

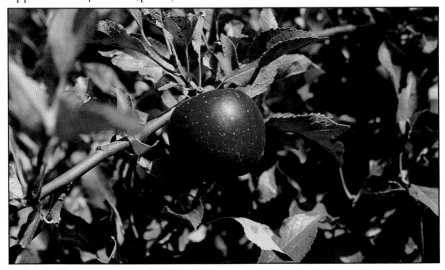

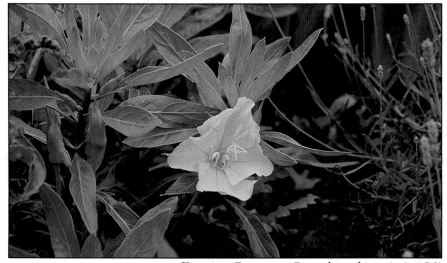

Evening Primrose *Oenothera biennis* (p. 86)

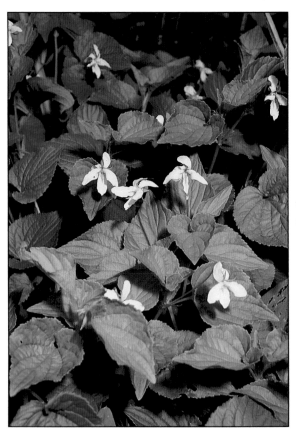

White Violet
*Viola canadensis* (p. 96)

Sassafras
*Sassafras albidum*
(p. 93)

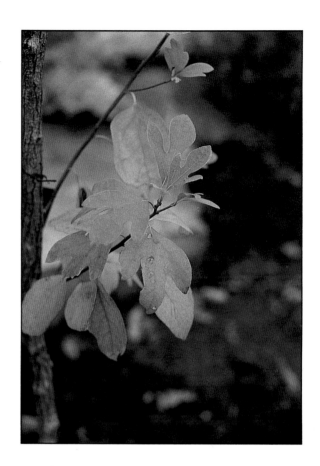

Hawthorn *Crataegus viridis* (p. 125)

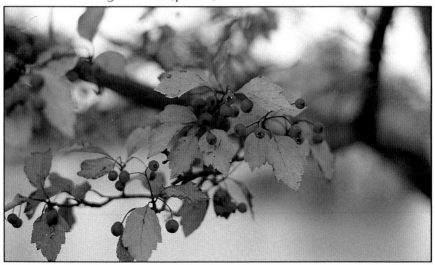

Hop
*Humulus lupulus*
(p. 111)

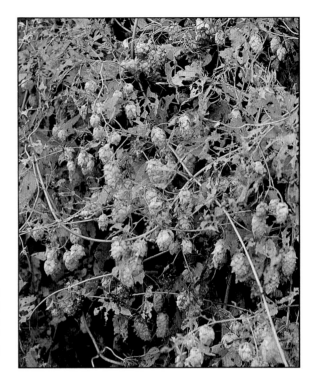

All herb species shown here have medicinal properties, but you should favor the species described in the "Tonic Herbs" chapters since they're the most effective.

Ginkgo   *Ginkgo biloba* (p. 88)

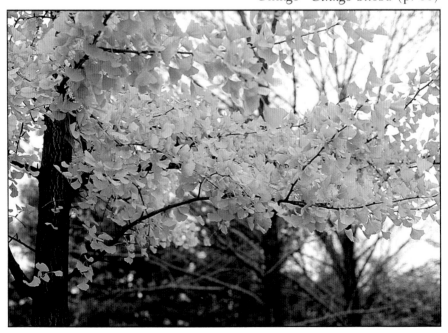

All photos by Amy Bridge

plant's growing habits firsthand. Of course, a few tonic herbs take several years before they're ready for harvest, but you can fall back on buying what you need while tending your little backyard plot. Most of what we term *wild* herbs are now commercially grown.

Growing your own supply of tonic herbs is very rewarding. When I first began growing herbs, I started with the scented varieties which I could use to scent my house in potpourris. From there, I went on to culinary varieties, and now I have several wild beds which contain herbs of tonic value. I have witch hazel shrubs, bayberry bushes, and a small stand of goldenseal in land that had been going to waste before. I feel good knowing that the land is not wasted and that it contains plants important for our future and perhaps for future generations. Some plants may become extinct if we do not make an obvious effort to save them, and what a loss it would be if they were to disappear. Even if you don't plan to use these plants, you could become a Johnny Herbseed of sorts by buying important seeds of healing plants to spread wherever you can (not violating any laws or property rights). It could make a difference to your children and grandchildren. I do this spring and fall, in addition to home crops I plant to use for myself and my family. It makes my heart full to know that some of these seeds will grow and bear fruit, passing on more seeds and spreading. Even if I don't see the results myself, the seeds represent a promise, a hope.

If you are thinking about cultivating your own plots to use, you can be assured a continuous supply of fresh material on hand whenever it is needed, without having to depend upon anyone else. You are thus assured of quality and freshness. Surprisingly, tonic herbs are the easiest to grow, and they often love to be neglected.

### Growing Wild

Most of the tonic herbs are plants we have relegated to the status of weeds. One of the main reasons they are so powerful is because we haven't bothered them much. Oh, we cuss and fuss over them when they pop up in places we don't want them, but we have basically left them alone. We haven't hybridized them, sprayed them with chemicals, or planted them in dead soil or soil full of alien chemicals. This is perhaps the most important message for growing your own. These herbs must be planted in soil which is alive, in which earthworms can survive. That means natural soil, soil which hasn't been treated but which has been enriched with compost.

### Compost

Compost is a symbol of rebirth—nature's way of providing continual renewal. As dead material collects on the ground, the dampened material begins to heat up. Then magically it is transformed into a rich, dark humus capable of giving life to new forms, feeding microorganisms, and making a soil most suitable to growing healthy plants. This is the natural way of making the soil fertile. We have often made the mistake of depleting our land by planting and harvesting, only taking and never giving back. The result is food that's almost useless nutritionally. Don't allow that to happen with your tonic herbs.

Composting is an art that is invaluable if you garden. Compost provides fertilizer for the garden to condition depleted soil. Merely throw your garbage into a pile, use a pitchfork to flip it once in a while to add oxygen, and watch it heat up. Throw on leaves, grass clippings, manure, or kitchen wastes. For city dwellers concerned about dogs digging into piles or complaints from neighbors, you can use containers, boxes, or bins. It takes time for the compost pile to become ready for use, often months, but if you add earthworms (purchased from ads in gardening publications and fed a little chicken mash), your compost can be ready within 60 days. There is also a trick called the 14-day method, which requires that you shred all material and turn it every 2 days. Check the many books and periodicals available. As more people become aware of the cycle of life in the plant world, we are dependent on the soil and its ability to sustain life. Let's hope composting and organic gardening will become a growing trend.

Once you have compost available, simply prepare a bed by tilling your area. Rake out clumps of grass until smooth. Then, throw on some compost and till it into the ground well. Next, plant the seed according to directions and weed occasionally. Many people do a little gardening every year, whether in a big garden to supply vegetable produce or a patio container with a few tomatoes or flowers. Gardening is gardening, and the medicinal herbs grow just like vegetables. You just have to familiarize yourself with the particular herb's needs.

### Harvesting

Soon it will come time for harvesting, and your job is to harvest the appropriate part of the plant you need, whether it's the leaves, roots, seeds, or flowers. Herbal leaves should be gathered at the stage just before the flower fades because that's when they're at their peak. Gather flowers immediately after they open completely. Both should be harvested on a clear, warm morning after the dew has dried. Gather one herb at a time, and either prepare your recipe immediately if using fresh plant material, or prepare to dry it.

To dry, place leaves, stems, or flowers in a single layer on cookie sheets or brown paper, and put them in a protected place out of the sun. It is important that this place be well ventilated. Drying will take several days, and you'll know the plants are dried when they crumble easily. Then, when the moisture is completely gone, the plant material can be placed in jars and stored.

For seeds, wait until they are fully mature to harvest. Cut the stem about 6 inches below the seed heads and bundle them to make a bouquet. Secure the stems with a rubber band. Tie a brown paper sack over the seed heads, and then hang them in a dark room. In several weeks they will be fully dry, and you'll see many seeds in the bottom of the sack. By rubbing the seed heads, you can loosen the remaining seeds. Clean out any debris, and place the seeds in an open bowl for another few days to make sure they are completely moisture free. Then place them in jars for storage.

Roots, barks, and twigs are another story. Twigs are usually collected in autumn, then dried in the open air. Barks can be collected in fall or early spring and oven dried or spread out to dry naturally. Only the inner bark of slippery elm is used. For rhizomes and roots, dig the plant carefully, making sure the root is not damaged. Roots and rhizomes should be harvested during the plant's dormant stage before growth or after the top has died back. This will ensure that the cells are full of sufficient food stores and nutrients—exactly what you want. Scrub the roots with a vegetable brush to remove the dirt. If the roots are thin they can be left whole. Large roots, however, should be sliced lengthwise and dried in a low-temperature oven until brittle or spread out in a layer to dry in the open air.

As always, check to make sure plant materials are completely dry before storing. If any moisture is left in the material, it will mold. If you discover mold, discard that batch and begin all over again. You always want your product to be fresh and free from contamination.

# Blood-Purifying Tonic Herbs
## To Cleanse Toxins from the Body

Blood-purifying tonic herbs cleanse toxins from the body. Cleansing the body of toxic material built up inside is perhaps the most important thing we can do. Nutritionist Jerry Deutsch at American Biologics in California, who has studied live-cell therapy and nutritional treatments for degenerative diseases like cancer and AIDS, insists this cleansing is a must. "It is possible to lock toxins within our bodies; so, if you wish to use nutrition-rich foods in a healing capacity, you have to make sure you detoxify. That would be the first step."

Herbalist Jude Williams agrees. "Getting rid of poisons within our bodies means we are one step ahead of the game. A clean body means a healthy body. Toxins can drag down our systems. Cleansing the poisons can help every organ in the body, but most especially the liver, which stores a great deal of the toxins we come in contact with."

But who needs to rid the body of accumulated toxic material? Today, just about all of us. If you smoke or are around smokers; if your eating has been nutritionally poor (fast foods, fried foods, too much meat, chemically treated foods); if you've worked in factories or with chemicals; or if you've been exposed to pollution in the water, soil, or air; then you've absorbed poisons into your body. These poisons can build up and lead to later problems in the form of minor illnesses or even life-threatening diseases.

Therefore, a cleansing and renewal program becomes necessary to flush out those toxins. Traditionally, a group of herbs called *blood cleansers* or *blood tonics* has been used for just this purpose. For the most part, each of these herbs has, in its own way, phytochemicals which cause it to act as a diuretic (increasing passage of urine) or a laxative, or to increase perspiration. All these methods help us wash accumulated toxins out of the body. Many herbalists recommend occasionally taking an internal bath as well as an external one.

Blood-cleansing tonics can do just that. They allow the impurities of living to be washed from our bodies easily and naturally so that good health shines through unimpeded. These blood-cleansing herbs can be used in a tonic or tea singly or in a combination health brew with several other herb types. These herbs also can be used as a prelude therapy intended to cleanse the body before taking another type of tonic to address more serious health problems. It's really up to you and how you feel. Do not use a cleansing tonic more than 3 days. If you really feel the need to do more cleansing, then rest 3 days, and begin again. But you don't want to tax your body.

Remember: tonics work slowly and gently on the system. There is no magic drink that can instantly transform you. These herbal tonics will indeed work if given a chance. Here are twelve types of the most favored blood-cleansing herbs and an explanation of what each does for the body. Knowing all this, you'll be able to choose a tonic appropriate to your needs.

# APPLE PECTIN

*Malus pumila*

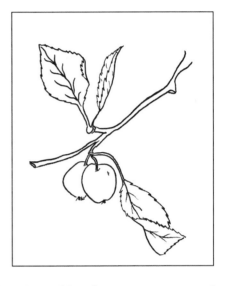

## REPORTED BENEFITS

"An apple a day keeps the doctor away." Nutritionists and herbalists still consider apples the most important of the blood cleansers. Apples contain high amounts of vitamin C, especially right under the skin, but more important, they contain pectin. In recent studies at the Michigan Cancer Foundation in Detroit, pectin found in certain fruits, including apples, blocked receptors on the surface of cancer cells. Pectin has also been found capable of removing unwanted metals and toxins, which makes it valuable in radiation therapy. Some have claimed that pectin can remove any trace of nuclear radiation. It also lowers cholesterol, helps gout, and reduces risk of heart disease and gallstones. If someone really wanted to remove poisons from the body, then this is how. Some people have even used apple pectin to pass job-related drug testing. That's how strongly it works.

Dr. Harold J. Reilly and Ruth H. Brod in *Edgar Cayce Handbook for Health Through Drugless Therapy* (1988) state, "Since most people are toxic to a greater or lesser degree, I have found that a good cleansing routine with the apple-diet regimen is the first step toward improving assimilation and elimination for anyone. If one is reasonably well, the detoxification will bring about an almost euphoric feeling of well-being . . . If one is not well, the apple-cleansing regimen is an excellent beginning of a therapeutic program." The Cayce apple diet they refer to involves eating only fresh apples for three days, drinking water or black coffee, and at the end of the third day, taking a dose of 2 tablespoons of olive oil. Cayce recommends such a regime for trance. I think the use of apple pectin in tonic form would accomplish the same goal.

## TONIC USAGE

Pectin occurs in ripe fruits, especially apples of all kinds. The apple with the greatest concentration of pectin is the crab apple, which is useful in making homemade jellies. Pectin is what causes the jelly to jell.

For tonics, make sure your apples—whatever kind you choose—are organically grown and free of pesticides. To prepare the apples, wash, core, and make thin slices, leaving skins on. If you use crab apples, merely wash and slice. Use a food dehydrator or spread a layer of slices on a cookie sheet and place it in a low oven (200° F) and dry until leathery but not crisp. Store in a closed glass jar. The apples will keep for a long time, but be sure to discard them after 1 year or if you get moisture into the jar and the product molds.

This will give you a concentrated source of pectin. To make the tonic, merely place 2 to 3 slices of the dried apples into a mug, and pour boiling water over them. Let steep for 3 to 5 minutes, then remove the slices, and drink. You should drink about 3 mugs a day. You won't need to add sweetener, since the tea is naturally sweet and tastes like hot apple juice. But if you wish, add a little honey. Do not add cream or milk. If you can fast during this time, apple pectin tea will cleanse the body all the better, and this is perhaps preferable if you continue a tonic therapy program. If fasting is not an option, then a light healthful diet is recommended, perhaps with nourishing soups and juices. Stay away from artificial sweeteners and chemical additives.

Feel free to use the pectin tonic when you feel the need. Apple pectin is also a good addition to a blend of several herbs. Since many herbs used for tonics are bitter, the sweet apple taste will help make these brews more palatable.

## AVAILABILITY

You can buy fresh organic apples at some farmers' markets and certain grocery stores, but make sure they're organic. Some mail-order firms deal in organic produce; you can ask for their catalogs.

Apple trees are also easy to grow if you have the space. You can also obtain the apple pectin in dried form at any health food store. Just add a couple of tablespoons to your teacup and cover with boiling water.

# BURDOCK

*Arctium lappa*
Also called great burdock or snake rhubarb
*Caution:* Make sure you are getting the true great burdock. The plant is often confused with other herbs that may be harmful and with common burdock, which has a hollow stem and little medicinal value.

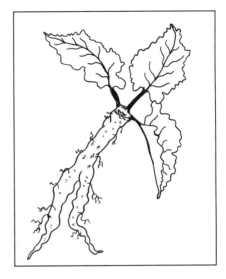

## REPORTED BENEFITS

Burdock, an ancient healing herb, has been called a pesty weed. Common to Europe and North America, it favors weedy roadsides and nitrogen-rich soil. As its name suggests, it has fruiting heads covered with burrs, but its leaves are dock shaped. The sturdy stem reminds one of rhubarb. Burdock is commercially cultivated in Japan as a vegetable, and in fact the roots have a mildly bitter potato-and-celerylike flavor.

In the past, its strong, hardy roots have been used in beer-making, but the Ojibwa (Chippewa) first used it as a "blood medicine." Burdock is also one of the four ingredients in the purported cancer remedy, Essiac, a recipe purportedly handed down from the Ojibwa. This root and sometimes the leaves were used by North American tribes as a stomach tonic. Today we find confirmation of its healing power. Researchers from Hungary have reported that burdock root contains antitumor properties, while Japanese researchers found reduced cell mutation in their experiments with it. Burdock has a mild laxative quality as well as being mildly diuretic and sweat-inducing. It is also good for the skin, soothing acne, psoriasis, and other skin disorders. As the Ojibwa found, it stimulates the digestive system and the liver and helps soothe ulcers. Two compounds have been found in the root which inhibit the growth of bacteria and fungi. These are especially concentrated in the fresh foot and can greatly benefit and renew the body's system, since they help resist infection.

## TONIC USAGE

The root of the burdock plant is most commonly used, fresh or dried (but fresh is usually thought best). You can harvest the root from first-year plants. Dig roots in the fall. Scrub them, then slice or chop them into thin, small pieces. To use the fresh root in tonic form, place 1 teaspoon of the root into a saucepan. Add 1 pint of water. Bring to a boil, then cover and reduce heat. Simmer for 20 minutes, cool until just warm, and strain. Drink 2 cups daily, perhaps adding a few herbs for taste, like dried parsley, a pinch of onion flakes, or a dash of fresh lemon juice. This brew really is quite tasty. Remember that you may feel worse before feeling better. This means old toxins are being released into the bloodstream before being flushed out. Soon after this, you should have a feeling of strength, well-being, and energy. To use the dried root, simply slice thinly and evenly, and place it in a good dehydrator or warm oven until brittle. Store in a closed container and use as described above. The dried root keeps indefinitely if stored from moisture.

## AVAILABILITY

Burdock is grown easily from seed. Sow seeds in early spring as soon as the soil has warmed up. The plant doesn't take well to transplanting because of its long taproots. It's best to prepare the beds with mounds of soft soil to make it easier to harvest the roots.

Burdock is also available commercially, dried, in health food stores. You may be able to obtain the fresh root at stores featuring ethnic foods, since the Japanese frequently use it in their cooking.

# CHICORY

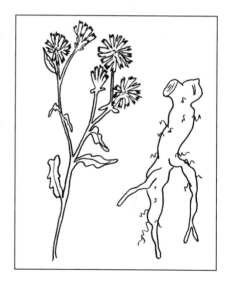

*Cichorium intybus*
Also called succory and witloof

## REPORTED BENEFITS

Chicory was a cultivated crop for thousands of years, which can be traced to the Egyptians, before it became a lowly roadside weed. Before it lost favor, chicory was an ingredient in many remedies. Queen Elizabeth I of England often consumed the broth of this plant. And Thomas Jefferson so loved the imported Italian seeds which soon grew into bright blue flowers that he hurriedly sent a note to his friend George Washington, explaining the virtues of chicory, calling it "one of the greatest acquisitions a farmer can have."

He didn't know how right he was. In 1940 a research project determined that two bitter substances within chicory act as sedatives on the central nervous system, and compounds found within the roasted root kill bacteria. Chicory is deemed a very safe, very mild tonic. As a blood cleanser it has laxative and diuretic properties, but it is especially associated with protecting the liver from excessive caffeine consumption. This is interesting, considering that in the early 20th century chicory root was used as a coffee substitute. It has also been said to increase bile flow, decrease inflammations, aid in jaundice, and lower cholesterol and blood sugar.

## TONIC USAGE
The fresh green chicory leaves and shoots have often been added to salads, creating a strong green flavor similar to that of dandelion. However, the root, fresh or dried, is most often used in tonics.

It is easy to make a bed of chicory in any corner of the yard or garden as long as you leave it alone to grow. Dig only the second-year roots since the first-year roots are quite small. Scrub and scrape; then slice thinly. Dry the root in a 325° F oven for 30 minutes until dark roasted or until it begins to smell like chocolate cake. Then, you know it's ready. Cool the chicory and then grind it with a mortar and pestle, or put it in a plastic bag and lightly smash it with a hammer. Store the roots in a closed container for future use. Use it somewhat as you would coffee: place 1 teaspoon of ground root in your cup, top it with boiling water, and let it steep a few minutes. If you don't want grounds in your cup, strain or tie the chicory root into a small bag using part of a coffee filter. Or use fill-it-yourself tea bags available where herb supplies are sold.

You will want to drink no more than 4 cups per day. The drink has a bittersweet taste which resembles coffee slightly. Drink plain.

## AVAILABILITY
Chicory is a common weed along roadsides, but don't use the wild plant growing there since it may be contaminated by poisons from car fumes, pesticide sprays, and more. It's best if you grow your own patch. Seeds can be obtained. You may find chicory coffee, but it will most likely be blended with other things, like regular coffee or dandelion.

# CLARY SAGE

*Salvia sclarea*
Also called clear eye, Christ's eye, and ramona

## REPORTED BENEFITS
Clary sage, a cleansing tonic herb, has a fragrant, balsamlike scent and a long history of medicinal uses. Its Latin name *salvia* means "health," and people have long revered plants of the sage family as a source of well-being.

Ancient Druids in Britain even tried to resuscitate the dead with sage in ritual ceremonies, such was the belief in the power of this family of herbs.

An erect biennial, clary sage is similar to garden sage but differs in composition. It grows 3 to 5 feet with heart-shaped broad leaves. The seeds have been used for centuries as an eyewash, hence its nickname *clear eye*. The seeds when moistened produce a mucilage which makes it easy to remove foreign matter from the eye. The herb is native to southern Europe and the Mediterranean; so, it prefers full sun and sandy, well-drained soil.

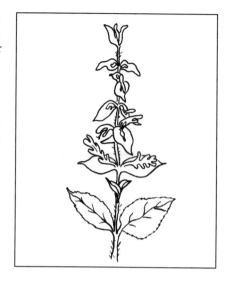

Commercially, the essential oil has been used as a flavoring in beverages, baked goods, puddings, candies, and liqueurs. Aromatherapists report that the essential oil causes euphoria and a marked relaxation response. It's a good idea to drink the tea in the evening before bed so that you don't fall asleep while driving or working. In the 16th century clary sage was added to wine to make it more potent. Interestingly, it has also been substituted for hops in beer-making. As for clary sage's healing attributes, it has been deemed an antispasmodic, an astringent, and a carminative. The antispasmodic properties come from nerol, found in the essential oil. Early herbalists used clary sage as a tea for digestive upsets and liver disorders and as a kidney tonic. Clary is also an antidepressant, diuretic, nervine, and sedative. Clary is good for painful menstruation and other female reproductive system problems. It can serve as an all-around tonic.

## TONIC USAGE

It is easy to grow clary sage if you have a small area with good drainage and full sun. Sow seed in spring. Once seedlings are developing well, thin to allow room for them to grow. The plants will flower in their second year, and after that they will self-sow. Divide them about every 3 years to avoid overcrowding.

You can harvest leaves in the fall of the first year, but for the strongest tonic, wait for the second year. Then you can harvest the flowering tops and leaves, since they contain the greatest concentration of essential oil within the plant.

Make a good, strong tea according to your taste, using fresh or dried plant material, perhaps 1 tablespoon of dried herb or 2 tablespoons of fresh herb to a teacup. Pour boiling water over the herb, cover, and let steep 10 to 20 minutes. Drink lukewarm, 1 or 2 cups at bedtime.

## AVAILABILITY
Clary sage is easy to grow yourself. Seeds can be obtained from mail-order herb companies. You can also order the dried herb.

# YELLOW DOCK

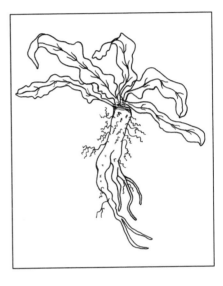

*Rumex crispus*

## REPORTED BENEFITS
As cleansing tonics go, yellow dock is high on the list. In Greece, dock was used as a purgative, and its name once meant "to cleanse." It has remained an important medicine since 500 B.C., and herbalists have long recommended the root as an astringent tonic and blood purifier. Yellow dock is a detoxifier, and the root decoction provides the minerals potassium, manganese, and iron, which are readily absorbed by the body. It outdoes spinach nutritionally, with a third more protein, iron, calcium, potassium, beta carotene, and phosphorus, and more than double the vitamin C. Because yellow dock is such a powerhouse of vitamins, it became an important vegetable during the Great Depression. This herb helps reduce swollen glands and inflammation. It also contains rumicin, a liver decongestant. Since liver disorders are often related to skin problems, it is also effective in treating skin discolorations related to liver disease, as well as eczema, psoriasis, skin cancer, and even leprosy. It stimulates the liver to produce bile. Yellow dock is a safe laxative that also strengthens the colon. Dr. Edwin R. Spencer in *All about Weeds* (1974) states, "The root has long been used in home remedies. It can be made into tonics, laxatives, and salves." This herb continues to be an important ingredient in alterative preparations, which alter or restore healthy bodily functions, in Germany, Russia, France, England, China, and other countries.

Many early North American tribes discovered the plant's amazing abilities. They applied compresses of crushed yellow-dock roots to cuts and boils. Physicians in earlier centuries used the roots as a laxative and a remedy for anemia, since the roots had the reputed ability to draw iron from the soil as they grew. European peasants used the leaves to avoid scurvy since they are very high in vitamin C. But be sure to exercise care when using the leaves since they are also high in oxalic acid, which can aggravate people with a tendency for gout.

## TONIC USAGE

Yellow dock is a weedy perennial with long carrot-shaped taproots, the inside of which is yellow or orange colored. The plant flowers June through August and is naturalized in North America. In early spring you can recognize yellow dock's long, narrow leaves with curly, wavy edges. In summer, this European perennial grows a flower stalk up to 5 feet tall. The stalk then soon becomes covered with dense clusters of tiny flowers, the flower giving way to seed clusters. One plant may contain as many as 40,000 seeds; so, you can see how determined this plant is to reproduce. The term *dock* suggests the European custom of removing part of the sheep's or dog's tail to dock it. All weeds were eventually called dock, since they were to be removed from sight. But this herb is difficult to remove, because if you pull or dig up a root, the slightest piece left in the ground will regrow. This is fine if you want to use the plant a lot. Today it grows as a weed that's hard to control, but what a power-packed weed it is. If you plan to grow it yourself, make sure you grow it in a contained area with plenty of sun. In spring sow the seed directly into your prepared bed.

Dig the yellow dock roots in late summer or autumn or in early spring, depending on how old the bed is. Give the roots one year to grow. Gently wash the root, then cut it in half lengthwise, and dry it in a cool, dark place or low oven.

For a tonic drink, use 1 teaspoon of the dried root in 1 cup of boiling water, cover, and steep for 30 minutes. Strain. The herb has a vegetable brothlike taste. Drink 1 to 2 cups a day. Be very cautious since you can overdose on this herb; symptoms include stomachache and nausea. Be sure you don't exceed the recommended dosage.

## AVAILABILITY

The plant is easy to grow or to find growing wild in fields near the beach, roadsides, and riverbanks coast to coast. Just make sure these areas are pesticide- and pollution-free.

Yellow dock is readily available at health food stores that carry dried herbs. Seeds can be bought from herb specialty catalogs.

# DANDELION

*Taraxacum officinale*

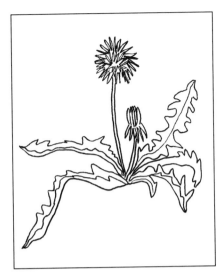

## REPORTED BENEFITS

Although the dandelion may be the most hated of the weeds, the plant is so good for you, it's hard to believe that so many people want to destroy it. Dandelion is higher in beta carotene than carrots, and it's also high in iron, calcium, potassium, phosphorus, zinc, and magnesium, as well as vitamins $B_1$, $B_2$, $B_5$, $B_6$, $B_{12}$, D, C, and E. The leaves have long been used for spring salads, sautéed and steamed. Dandelion has been a favorite traditional spring tonic. In the 10th century, Arabian physicians recognized that dandelion increased urine production; so, they considered it a tonic and mild laxative. In Europe the herb gained a reputation as a liver remedy. American colonists took to it quickly. Dandelion was incorporated as a diuretic in the *U.S. Pharmacopoeia* from 1831 to 1926. This root was also an ingredient in Lydia E. Pinkham's Vegetable Compound, a popular 19th century patent medicine for menstrual discomforts, probably resulting from its diuretic and antiinflammatory properties. Humans and beasts both need green things in the spring, old herbals state. A revitalization of blood was necessary to the system for cleansing. Dr. Salmon's *The Family Dictionary* (1710), an old herbal, refers to spring tonics as *sallets. Acetaria: A Discourse on Sallets* (1699) includes many listings of common and uncommon herbs. Dandelion was always included. The Chinese have long revered the yellow flower, considering it one of their six most important medicinal herbs. They have prescribed the whole plant for over 1,000 years for colds, pneumonia, hepatitis, boils, and ulcers. They've also used a poultice of chopped dandelion to treat breast cancer. India's ayurvedic physicians did the same.

Current research shows that the plant oils do have a stimulating effect on the body, strengthening the whole system as well as the liver and gallbladder. They promote the flow of bile, reduce inflammation of the bile duct, and help eliminate gallstones. The oils are also good for chronic hepatitis, since they reduce jaundice and swelling of the liver. Dandelion absorbs toxins from the body, regulating intestinal bacteria, and some studies have suggested that it helps prevent cancer. This gentle diuretic won't deplete the body of nutrients and minerals, since it is so packed with vitamins that it replaces any flushed away and then some. Dandelion contains 14,000 IU of vitamin A, compared with the carrot's 11,000. It is also rich in another antioxidant, vitamin C. Both vitamins A and C help prevent cell damage, which scientists say is helpful in preventing certain cancers. The American Cancer Society recommends a diet high in antioxidant nutrients to help prevent several cancers, particularly colon cancer. Another study has shown that dandelion also inhibits the growth of fungus implicated in vaginal yeast infections. Japanese studies point to its tumor-inhibiting activity, as well as its value in helping arthritis. The herb is recommended for people under stress or who feel internally sluggish, as well as for people who are sedentary or overweight. It helps the bladder and stomach, although people with an irritable stomach or bowel or with acute inflammations are cautioned against using it. Dandelion has been indicated for adult-onset diabetes because the root's inulin doesn't tax the pancreas the way refined sugars do.

The root has long been thought of as helpful for strengthening anyone with a run-down immune system. Herbalists say it is one of the best herbs for "building up the blood."

Almost everyone has seen the perennial herbaceous plant, with its lance-shaped leaves and bright yellow buttonlike flowers. The French called this plant *dent de lion* or "lion's tooth." Dandelion adapts well and was introduced to North America from Europe to provide food for honeybees in early spring. Now the plant grows worldwide.

## TONIC USAGE

The roots can be roasted and used as a coffee substitute, often mixed with chicory. (Follow the same roasting directions used for chicory in this chapter.) You can make a tea of the leaves or root, as you wish. The leaves make a green, bitter tea, while the roasted root is bitter and coffeelike. Dandelion is safe to drink as much as you like but the recommended maximum is usually 3 cups per day. For dandelion tea, gather young, tender leaves in early spring. Place 2 tablespoons of fresh leaves or 1 tablespoon of dried leaves into 1 cup of boiling water. Cover, steep 10 minutes, strain, and drink.

For a root drink that's more coffeelike, pour boiling water over 2 to 3 teaspoons of powdered dandelion root per cup of water, and steep 15 minutes. Strain and enjoy.

## AVAILABILITY

Gather dandelion from yards and fields free of pesticides and lawn chemicals. Some wild seed catalogs now carry dandelion. You can also visit some groceries and farmers' markets in early spring when they may have fresh greens.

# FENNEL

*Foeniculum vulgare*

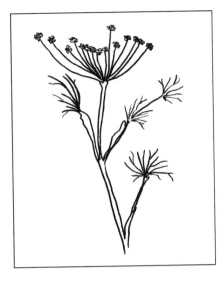

## REPORTED BENEFITS

Nicholas Culpeper's English herbal of 1649, which outlined herbs' medicinal uses, claimed that fennel helped inhibit kidney stones, prevented nausea and gout, and cleared the liver and lungs. The tea was used to cure colic in babies, and when gargled it served as a breath freshener. Fennel is a weak diuretic and a mild stimulant which also soothes the stomach. Herbalists have used fennel cooked as a broth and as a slimming remedy. It is considered a tonic and a digestive aid. Fennel root is considered the best of the five great aperitive roots; its juice taken on an empty stomach is great for fevers, as a sleep agent, and for reducing gas. The leaves taken in a decoction are said to strengthen vision. The dried seed has been used in liqueurs and medicines.

The Greeks used fennel to treat over twenty illnesses, and reduced appetite is again a side effect mentioned in connection with fennel. The plant has a main taproot similar to the carrot's except that it is white. Fennel has a strong, pleasing odor.

## TONIC USAGE

Fennel is a semihardy perennial. Seed can be easily sown in late fall or early spring. Harvest seeds when they turn yellowish green to brown. Snip the seed heads, place them in paper bags, and store them in a warm, dark place to dry. Once dry, place the seed heads in jars for year-round use. You can use the leaves, seeds, or roots as you wish. The roots, however, are considered the strongest of the three for use in tonics. Fennel has a delicate aniselike taste.

Use 1 tablespoon of dried or 2 tablespoons of fresh material to 1 cup of boiling water. Cover and let steep 10 minutes. Strain. Drink lukewarm, up to 3 cups per day.

## AVAILABILITY

Fennel is readily available at health food stores which sell dried herbs. Seed for eating, fresh leaves, and stalks can be purchased at specialty groceries. The plant is easy to grow. Seeds are widely available.

# LICORICE ROOT

*Glycyrrhiza glabra*

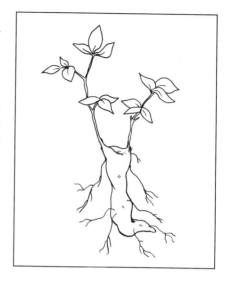

## REPORTED BENEFITS

Like its name, licorice root has the characteristic licorice taste that makes it an easy tonic to take and one that's good to blend with a more bitter brew. The herb is fifty times sweeter than sugar. A hardy perennial with a stringy taproot, brown on the outside and yellow in the inside, it grows to 4 feet tall. With many offshoots, the root is a tangled mess. It is extensively cultivated worldwide in Russia, Greece, Spain, the United States, Canada, Australia, and other places. It flowers in midsummer and resembles the sweet pea. It was once used as a candy flavoring, but now anise has practically replaced it.

The root was mentioned in the first Chinese herbal. The Chinese called it the great detoxifier. Licorice root was recommended for soothing sore throats, urinary and bowel disorders, and for helping clear respiratory passages. Licorice root has also been used as an antispasmodic, a mild laxative, and a cough remedy. It has diuretic action, eases ulcers, and reduces arthritis inflammation by ridding the body of toxins.

As if that were not enough, the root extract produces mild estrogenlike effects; so, it's helpful for women who have menstrual problems or who are in menopause. This estrogenic activity has clearly been established in an animal study. In another study, women who could not ovulate were able to have normal ovulation after using the extract.

Other studies, conducted by the Japanese, have shown that licorice root modulates and strengthens the activity of other herbs. Its status as a tonic is probably due to the cumulative effect of all its medicinal properties. It is very complex. Licorice root adjusts concentrations of blood salts, stimulating and sustaining proper adrenal function. Licorice root protects the body's own detoxification plant, the liver, from such diseases as cirrhosis and hepatitis. Studies have also proved that the chemical glycyrrhizin contained in licorice reduces cancer tumors in rats and has even killed off HIV cells before they turned into full-blown AIDS.

A group of Russian researchers has found that licorice root inhibits tumor growth (sarcoma-45 and Ehrlich ascites cells). Another recent study has found that licorice root actually stimulates the production of interferon, a chemical critical to enhancing the immune system, which has proven key to preventing and treating many immune-response deficiency diseases, AIDS included. A physician at Sloan-Kettering in New York stated that phytochemicals (essential oils in plants containing the healing chemicals) are extremely effective in combating growth and development of cancer cells, specifically for prostate and breast cancers. Licorice root is a natural disease fighter with strong antibacterial and antifungal properties.

## TONIC USAGE
If one overdoses on licorice root, it can produce the opposite effect, causing salt and water retention. For this reason, cardiac patients, people with high blood pressure or kidney disorders, pregnant women, and people who are very overweight should carefully monitor their intake.

You can take root cuttings to get licorice root started. Growth is slow the first 2 years. Harvest only 3- to 4-year-old roots. Dig the roots but leave remnants to regrow and continue your bed. Cut the root in pieces and dry it completely. Licorice root has a sweet, somewhat rooty taste.

For licorice root tea, bring water to a boil and lower heat. Add 1 tablespoon of dried root per cup and simmer covered for 10 minutes. Strain and cool. Drink 1 to 2 cups per day. If more cleansing is needed, rest 3 days, then repeat.

## AVAILABILITY
You can buy licorice root extract in health food stores by the ounce. The dried root is also available. The plant is easy to grow, but it takes at least 3 years before you'll be able to use it medicinally.

# OREGON GRAPE

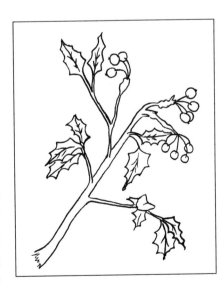

*Mahonia aquifolium*
Also called mountain grape and holly barberry

## REPORTED BENEFITS
Oregon grape, the state flower of Oregon, was very popular in the 1800s as a medicine and food. The ailments Oregon grape is said to help include kidney disorders, skin problems, heartburn, and more. One tonic required soaking the roots in warmed beer to cure jaundice. Oregon grape appeared on the market in the late

1800s and was listed in official pharmacopoeias until 1950. Europeans have always considered it an excellent blood purifier.

Dr. Edward E. Shook in *Advanced Treatise in Herbology* found Oregon grape an exceptional tonic and laxative that's helpful for the liver and digestive complaints. He states that it is an excellent nerve tonic.

Oregon grape has direct action on the skin, unlike any other herb. It actually restores skin to a clear condition following a skin disease or other illness that may cause the complexion to dry out or become ulcerated. It is a good source for berberine, an active substance in goldenseal and barberry. This hollylike plant grows on the east coast of North America and throughout the Pacific Northwest. It is important to liver health. Studies show that it stimulates bile production, enhancing liver function and getting rid of system sluggishness. It is an alterative herb. However, people who have been overeating or eating rich food should use a gentler blood cleanser, like dandelion or apple pectin.

## TONIC USAGE

Oregon grape makes a strong laxative, tonic, and skin cleanser. It's especially well suited to be combined with dandelion root. But since Oregon grape root has a bitter taste, it's best to combine it with sweet herbs to help it go down better. Although the root or rhizome is used medicinally, the deep purple berries (not really grapes) can be made into jams, jellies, juices, or syrups.

You can propagate the plant with seeds collected from the berries in fall, and use suckers, layers, or cuttings taken in midsummer. Oregon grape is a spring-blooming evergreen shrub with fragrant yellow blooms. It grows 3 feet high. The shrub grows especially well under pine trees and is very attractive.

You can obtain the root from second-year plants, making sure you leave some of the rhizome behind to self-propagate. Slice and dry well. To make an infusion, use 1 ounce of dried root and place it in boiling water. Let simmer covered for 30 minutes. Strain, cool, and bottle, placing it in the refrigerator. Take 2 to 3 tablespoons of this per day. Since the fruit is high in vitamin C, you could add it to your tea for added benefit.

## AVAILABILITY

Oregon grape is easy to grow. Seeds and plants are available at nurseries. The dried root can be found in most health food stores which sell dried herbs.

# RHUBARB

*Rheum rhabarbarum*

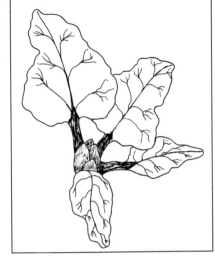

## REPORTED BENEFITS

Rhubarb, originally found in Siberia, has spread throughout the world. Traders on camel caravans brought it to Greece and Rome. Rhubarb not only tastes good; it's also a good tonic. It has served as a famous spring tonic after a long, harsh winter. American colonists valued it as a vegetable that could be eaten as fruit, and it was also easy to grow.

Rhubarb contains vitamins A and C, calcium, and other nutrients. It is a brisk laxative that's good for the stomach and cleanses the bowels without producing a rebound effect of constipation. Although it can remove irritating substances in the bowels, its astringent quality assures that the diarrhea does not become severe. Rhubarb is also a blood purifier. Turkey rhubarb (*Rheum palmatum*) comes from China and East India, and this type of rhubarb is used in the Essiac cancer remedy. American garden rhubarb and Turkey rhubarb strongly resemble each other, but the latter is much larger.

## TONIC USAGE

Rhubarb, pretty much trouble-free, will grow anywhere. The cold produces the delicate pink on the stalks, and it is this part that's used to make pies. The leaves, however, are *poisonous*. You can propagate this vegetable herb by division of the fleshy roots.

For a medicinal tea, use the dried rhizome, stripped of bark. You can powder the dried root in a grinder. Take 1 ounce of rhubarb root. Place it in 1½ pints of boiling water. Reduce heat and let simmer, covered, for 20 minutes. Strain, cool, and refrigerate. Take ¼ cup three times a day after light meals.

## AVAILABILITY

The fleshy roots can be divided. Rhubarb is readily available at nurseries or seed companies. A friend can give you a start, but each piece should have a good eye.

# SARSAPARILLA

*Smilax officinalis*

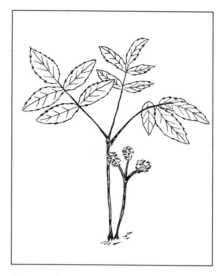

## REPORTED BENEFITS

Sarsaparilla has been the base for many 19th century tonics in the United States and Canada. Shakers, who healed with many herbs, grew and used sarsaparilla. The Shaker tonic Corbett's Compound Concentrated Syrup of Sarsaparilla was their most popular tonic, and many imitators sold similar syrups as elixirs. At first, sarsaparilla syrup was made with roots imported from Central and South America. Later, wild American sarsaparilla, *Aralia nudicaulis*, was used.

Native Americans used wild sarsaparilla to make a soothing, perspiration-inducing tea that helped heal burns, quiet coughs, reduce hypertension, and relieve symptoms of rheumatism, gout, and skin diseases.

Apparently, the root has many important functions in healing. One Chinese clinical study found a 90 percent degree effectiveness against primary syphilis. Several other studies verified the presence of antibiotic properties. The root actually attacks microbes in the bloodstream and neutralizes them. It has been used in the United States and China for rheumatism, arthritis, skin diseases, fevers, and digestive disorders. Sarsaparilla acts as a strong diuretic that stimulates excretion of wastes, such as uric acid and excess chloride. It promotes sweating action, thereby removing still more toxins from the lymphatic and circulatory systems.

## TONIC USAGE

Sarsaparilla has a mild root beer taste. The herb is very refreshing and fragrant and makes a dark, reddish tea. It is an evergreen woody vine which grows wild in the tropical forests of Mexico, Jamaica, and Central America. The wild American sarsaparilla is a native subshrub also called bristly sarsaparilla, which grows 1 to 3 feet, sending up suckers. It thrives in any good soil. Propagation is by seeds, root cuttings, or suckers. The bark of the wild American sarsaparilla can be used; dig the root in autumn.

To make a strong tea, place 2 teaspoons of crushed, fresh root or bark or 1 teaspoon of dried, powdered root in 1 cup of boiling water. Cover and steep 10 to 15 minutes. Strain and cool. Drink no more than 1 to 2 cups per day.

## AVAILABILITY

Sarsaparilla may be hard to obtain.

# SWEET WOODRUFF

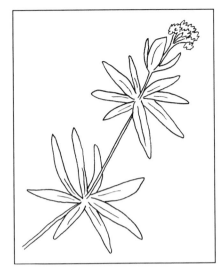

*Galium odoratum*
Also called master of the woods, mothherb, and woodward

## REPORTED BENEFITS

As its name implies, *sweet woodruff* is a sweet package rolled into one herb. Not only is the herb considered medicinal, but it is aromatic with an unusual vanillalike scent—but only when dried. And it has had culinary uses.

This low, spreading plant forms clumps 8 inches high with small, pretty white flowers. It loves to grow in shady spots and with its decorative qualities, almost anyone can keep sweet woodruff around.

The plant has spokelike leaf patterns which some have compared with paper ruffs used to decorate poultry. In the 14th and 15th centuries, it was used for scenting perfume. The Germans have used sweet woodruff to flavor their May wine, which was used as a tonic. May wine was featured since the 13th century in May Day celebrations greeting spring. They called the herb "master of the forest." Through the centuries, this herb has also been chopped and dried to flavor punches and fresh fruits and to make jellies and glazes for chicken and venison.

But what about its healing value? Herbalist Jude Williams, in *Jude's Herbal Home Remedies* (1992), states that sweet woodruff is good for liver disorders, cuts, and wounds; it also regulates heart activity. It is a diuretic and an antispasmodic. The herb has also been used as a blood purifier and tonic. It cleanses kidney and bladder obstructions, particularly stones, and relieves liver congestion and gallbladder difficulties. It has even been cited as a good herb for people with insomnia.

## TONIC USAGE

You can plant seeds in the fall or divide roots in the spring to get a good start. After sweet woodruff is established, it spreads quickly. Harvest in the spring right after it flowers. Let it dry in a cool, shady place. As it dries, you'll notice a marked vanillalike aroma. This comes from the chemical coumarin contained within the plant. Coumarin has been used in certain medications to thin the blood. Use cautiously and sparingly since it can cause hemorrhaging.

To make a healing tea, take 2 teaspoons of the dried material and add to 1 cup of boiling water. The tea has a mild, sweet, musky taste. Cover and let cool to room temperature. Limit intake to 1 cup per day, spread throughout the day.

## AVAILABILITY
You can easily grow sweet woodruff, and seed can be obtained through most seed and herb companies. It grows wild in wooded locations.

# Strengthening Tonic Herbs
## *To Help Build Up the Immune System*

All of us are waging a daily war we may be unaware of that does not concern land, money, politics, or religion. Every day, our bodies fight against invading bacteria, viruses, and numerous diseases that can damage or ultimately destroy us. And the weapon? The immune system. It's capable of producing antibodies that can distinguish between good (our own) and bad (invading or foreign) cells. This is indeed a miraculous system. We fight off invaders daily which never even penetrate the skin; so, we really do not know how many times an illness has been thwarted. It is only when the immune system has been weakened that it can be overpowered and we become ill.

But that's usually when we begin to worry, after the fact. Most health-care systems here and abroad act only after illness strikes. Sometimes what they offer is too little, too late. What if we were to invest in an alternate approach and take action to actually prevent illness. Then, we could sidestep pain and illness and trips to hospitals or physicians' offices. How much happier, simpler, and cheaper that would be. Apparently, many people are beginning to believe this is the best approach. Many health organizations, medical schools, and health insurers are beginning to focus attention on prevention instead of treatment. In the United States, Canada, France, and other countries national cancer institutes have suggested guidelines for diet and health. In 1989 two pharmaceutical firms introduced a new "drug" to help reverse and prevent an eye disease thought to be age related. But this supposed drug was simply a combination of nutrients.

Most modern studies confirm the benefits of improved nutrition. "A healthy immune system should be maintained at all times to prevent disease," an Ohio holistic health consultant, Joyce Frederick, insists. "We weaken the immune system by the consumption of chemical drugs and antibiotics, and we can rebuild it only by eating healthy foods, taking natural supplements and herbs, homeopathy, exercise, clean water, air, and sunshine. Immune-strengthening herbs stimulate and increase metabolic function."

So, if we intend to strengthen the body, we should make sure that the body is rested and cleansed of toxins. And it would be advisable to use tonic herbs high in vitamins, minerals, and other nutrients to boost our immune system and other systems in the body. Here are eight herbs proven to help us do just that.

# CALENDULA

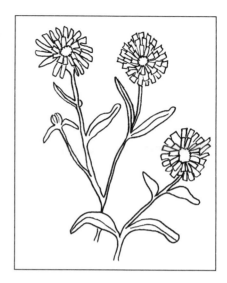

*Calendula officinalis*
Also called pot marigold

## REPORTED BENEFITS

It is hard to believe that a sunny yellow flower can be so important as a strengthener, but calendula has been deemed a useful medicinal since ancient times. It was used in the Mediterranean by ancient Greeks and known to Indian and Arabic cultures well before then. Shakespeare called calendula "herb of the sun" in *A Winter's Tale*, since the flowers open in the morning and close as the sun goes down.

An annual with large yellow or orange flowering heads, calendula grows throughout the world, where it is widely cultivated.

Calendula, commonly called pot marigold, contains a bitter yellow oil which is composed of fat, resin, sugar, potassium chloride, potassium sulfate, and sodium as well as bassora gum. The herb has reportedly eased the pain of cancer and checked its growth. The herb is antiinflammatory, antiseptic, and capable of healing wounds. Good for liver ailments, it was once commonly found on home medicine shelves. For centuries, the English and Germans believed that eating calendula flowers maintained health throughout the winter.

It aids bile secretion, and it is specifically useful in inflamed lymphatic nodes, duodenal ulcers, and some inflammatory skin lesions. Applied externally, the herb helps heal burns. This ability to accelerate healing makes it a stimulant that's helpful to the immune system. Laboratory studies show that calendula kills bacteria and fungi. It is a remedy against *candida* and gentle enough for applying to thrush (caused by *candida*) in children's mouths. The herb promotes the draining of swollen lymph glands. Modern herbalists have reported that it inhibits tumors and has been used successfully in treating abnormal cervical cells.

## TONIC USAGE

Gather calendula flower petals right after the plant blooms on a bright, sunny day. Dry them in a shady area on newspaper. When fully dry, be sure to store them in a tightly closed container.

Plant seeds in full sun, and it will flower from July to late fall.

Calendula tea has a pasty sweet taste with a salty aftertaste. Add 1 teaspoon of dried flowers or 2 teaspoons of fresh flowers to 1 cup of boiling water, cover, and steep 10 minutes. Drink 3 to 4 cups per day.

## AVAILABILITY
Calendula is readily available. It's also easy to grow; seeds can be purchased through nurseries and catalogs.

# COMFREY

*Symphytum officinale*
Also called knitbone, boneset, and healing herb

## REPORTED BENEFITS
Comfrey has received much attention for its ability to renew cells. The herb's medicinal qualities come from its production of allantoin and high amounts of protein. Certain varieties of comfrey contain almost 35 percent protein, equal to that of soybeans. Comfrey is also the only land plant to provide vitamin $B_{12}$. It is also high in 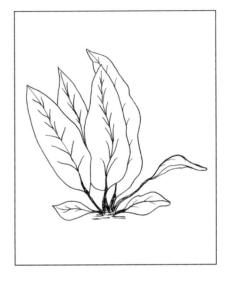 calcium, phosphorus, potassium, and trace minerals, and well as vitamins A and C.

Comfrey has been an important animal food source, especially in Africa, and an Englishman promoted its use as fodder in the late 19th century. North American homesteaders used it as winter feed for chickens since it is so packed with nourishment.

The word *comfrey* comes from the Latin *conferva* meaning "to boil, grow together, heal," in reference to its healing power. Comfrey repairs cells and digestive tract linings and acts as an astringent, demulcent, and weak sedative. Native to Europe and Asia, it has been naturalized elsewhere and was once the main herb for healing fractures and broken bones.

Studies show that comfrey inhibits prostaglandins, which can cause inflammation of the stomach lining. It has also been used to treat a variety of respiratory diseases. Although one study reported that rats fed a diet of 33 percent comfrey developed liver cancer, that amount of comfrey would be difficult for humans to consume. This study, however, suggests that large amounts of allantoin are unnecessary and may actually cause the opposite effect on health. But other studies prove its effectiveness in preventing cancer. In a 1965 study, water extracts of comfrey leaves were found to decrease tumor growth and increase survival time for cancer patients.

Dr. Charles J. Macalister, an English physician who studied the effects of comfrey in 1936, wrote about his findings. The blood counts of patients given doses of the herb had increased disease-fighting white blood cells (which demonstrates an increase in immune function) as much as 83 percent higher than those of patients not receiving the herb. English folk medicine also insists that comfrey is a cancer fighter.

## TONIC USAGE

As a perennial, comfrey grows very easily, and it does grow wild although it can make a beautiful specimen in a garden or flower bed, with its dark green fuzzy leaves growing up to 3 feet. A member of the borage family, comfrey has creamy yellow or purplish blue flowers. It is hardy and continues to grow even sometimes after frost. Comfrey is hard to get rid of since it can grow if even the slightest piece of root is left in the ground. You can use the roots or leaves, but it's probably best to use young leaves since they will contain less concentrations of allantoin.

Comfrey tea has a pleasant green, slightly bitter taste. Pour 1 cup of boiling water over 1 teaspoon of dried leaves or 3 teaspoons of fresh leaves and steep, covered, for 15 to 20 minutes. Strain. Drink 1 to 2 cups per day.

## AVAILABILITY

Comfrey propagation is by root division, and it is easy to grow if you have space. You can still purchase comfrey seed or roots through specialty catalogs. It may be hard to find, although some mail-order companies do sell it.

# ECHINACEA

*Echinacea purpurea*
Also called purple coneflower

## REPORTED BENEFITS

Native Americans used echinacea for many of their most tenacious sicknesses. American Plains tribes used various species to treat sore throats, toothaches, infections, wounds, skin problems, and infectious diseases such as mumps and smallpox, and even the rare case of cancer. These tribes simply sucked on the root, and samples of echinacea have been uncovered from campsites dating from the 1600s. In the late 19th century, H. C. F. Meyer patented a tonic made of echinacea and the herb was a top seller until the advent of modern medicine, when many herbs were cast aside. However, its popularity is again rising and since the mid-1930s, over 300 scientific articles have been written about it. Herbalists today debate over which is the most effective species, but the area in which it grows and the soil content probably make the biggest difference. Differences between species are probably negligible.

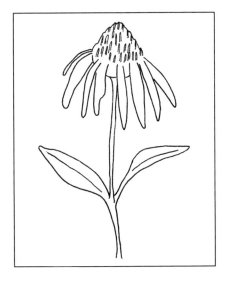

The U.S. Dispensatory stated more than 100 years ago that echinacea tincture increased resistance to infection, and their findings appear to be supported today. Echinacea is considered an alterative, an herb that alters the system and encourages health. It is also deemed a blood purifier. Studies have indicated that it is a powerful immune stimulant that increases chances of fighting off almost any disease. So far, it has been found to be completely safe. Clinical studies show that extracts of this herb improve white-blood-cell count and create other immune responses not completely understood. These qualities make echinacea an important strengthening herb.

Echinacea also stops bacteria that make cells susceptible to infection, and it is a natural, mild antibiotic that's effective enough to fight strep and staph infection. A study done with 200 children found that the group taking it had fewer illnesses, including respiratory and viral infections.

In the newsletter Health & Healing: Tomorrow's Medicine Today (December 1994) Dr. Julian Whitaker, a health practitioner and advocate of healthy nontoxic lifestyles, agreed with many herbalists on the importance of echinacea as a medicinal. He considers it a potent immune-system stimulant, and it is commonly prescribed in Europe. But Dr. Whitaker stresses that it should not be taken indefinitely, as body response diminishes over time. According to Arkansas herbalist Steven Foster in Echinacea: Nature's Immune Enhancer (1991), this herb was the most widely used remedy in America until the 1920s, when the discovery of penicillin and antibiotics replaced it. One German study found immune function, measured by one class of white blood cells, was boosted 120 percent within 5 days of use. Echinacea has been deemed a wonder herb.

## TONIC USAGE

Echinacea, a perennial which enjoys full sun, blooms July through fall. However, it takes 3 to 4 years to develop enough roots for a medicinal harvest. After the plant dies back in the late fall, dig the root. Then slice and dry the root for powdered use. Replant the crown after the root is harvested to continue your supply.

The tea is a bitter-tasting but slightly sweet brew, which tingles the tongue. Use 4 tablespoons of powdered root per quart of water. Simmer this over low heat, covered for 20 minutes, then strain. You can drink the tea hot or cool, 1 to 2 cups per day. Drink it 2 weeks on, 1 week off, and repeat the cycle if needed. But be sure to rest between dosage programs to keep the body from diminishing in response. Echinacea, however, cannot repair severely damaged immune systems, such as those with advanced AIDS or cancer.

## AVAILABILITY

The powdered root is available at some health food stores. Although echinacea is easy to grow, it requires a 3- to 4-year wait. Someone who wanted to use it immediately would have to buy it.

## ELECAMPANE

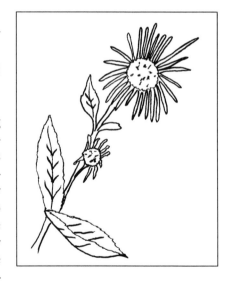

*Inula helenium*
Also called scabwort and horseheal

### REPORTED BENEFITS

Elecampane is often found growing near the ruins of European monasteries where monks cultivated it for its ability to help skin and bronchial disorders. The monks studied it closely and found that it had the ability to sustain the spirits. In fact, elecampane has been a medicinal recognized by herbalists from ancient times to the present. Among its ancient proponents are Dioscorides, Pliny, and Gerard. Culpeper called it priceless in healing virtues. Elecampane was also used to heal animals, specifically sheep and horses with skin and breathing disorders, hence its names *horseheal* or *scabwort*.

In discussing strengthening herbs, an important part of health is in the body's ability not only to be well nourished by vitamins and minerals, but also to be able to breathe adequately so that the blood can receive enough oxygen to nourish cells properly. In aiding these needs, elecampane is unbeatable. Experiments conducted in 1885 found that the active, bitter principle within the plant, *helenin*, was a powerful antiseptic and bactericide, killing ordinary bacteria, but in particular, the tuberculosis bacillus *Myobacterium tuberculosis*. So, it was used specifically for tuberculosis as well as for other respiratory problems, like asthma and bronchitis. In the 16th century, Spaniards used this amazing plant as a surgical dressing and they have deemed it an alterative tonic for the whole body. Elecampane was thought to improve general well-being, and the root increases one's appetite and promotes good digestion. It is also good for anemia. Europeans still sip cordials made with the infused root for this purpose. While Europeans favor using the root, the Chinese prefer using the flowers in the treatment of certain types of cancer. The herb contains sodium phosphate, which cleanses the liver and digestive organs. It also contains calcium chloride, which is good for the heart muscle.

## TONIC USAGE
This herb has nearly always been mixed with one or several healing herbs, possibly because of its bittersweet camphorlike flavor. Elecampane is fine to use by itself, especially if you find yourself with a weak lung condition.

This tall herb has daisylike flowers. The roots are light gray and hard, growing from a crown. A perennial, elecampane grows in full sun or semi-shade and blooms from spring to fall. Divide roots on 2-year plants or start it from seed. For serious medicinal use, use the 2-year-old roots. However, the leaves and stems can also be used to make a tea, although herbalists say the brew will not be as effective.

To make your tea, take ¼ cup of chopped root, add 1 pint of water, and bring to a boil. Cover, reduce heat, and simmer for 20 minutes. Cool and strain. Drink a small cup twice a day.

## AVAILABILITY
Elecampane can be found at some health food stores which sell dried herbs. It is easily grown.

# FENUGREEK

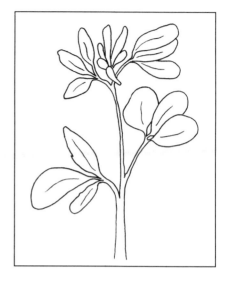

*Trigonella foenum-graecum*
Also called bird's foot and Greek hay-
seed

## REPORTED BENEFITS
Fenugreek, one of the oldest known
medicinal plants, dates from Egyptian times, when it was believed to
strengthen those recovering from illnesses. Like elecampane, it is also
good for bronchitis, but it also proves
good for colds and fevers.

In Greece, pregnant women were
given the boiled seeds mixed with
honey in the belief that fenugreek seeds gave them strength. In the Middle
East they have a special greeting for this herb they call *helbah*: "May you
tread in peace on the soil where it gave new strength and fearless mood to
gladiators, fierce and rude; helbah grows." Fenugreek is an important food
source in North Africa, where flour of the crushed seed is used to increase
weight, since the herb contains 25 percent protein. It also helps improve
protein utilization and inhibits phosphorus secretion. It has often been
thought of as an energizer and was an ingredient in Lydia Pinkham's popular health tonic.

Research has proven that the seed contain 30 percent mucilage, making
it a good laxative. It is also an expectorant and it helps relieve anemia,
diabetes, and ulcers. Clinical studies show it reduces both blood sugar and
cholesterol levels in animals. It contains a hormonelike substance similar to
that of the wild yam, which closely matches human sex hormones. For this
reason, in China it has been given to men to correct impotence and increase fertility, and to women to reduce menopausal symptoms and as a
calcium source.

## TONIC USAGE
This annual resembles sweet clover, except it has yellow, richly scented
flowers which bloom in early summer, followed by seed pods rich in minerals with a chemical composition close to that of cod liver oil.

Fenugreek's taste is pleasant and slightly bitter, with a hint of vanilla or
maple. Use the seeds or leaves. To make a tea, use 1 teaspoon of dried leaves
or 3 teaspoons of fresh leaves to 1 cup of water. Pour boiling water over the
leaves and let steep 10 minutes. Strain. Drink up to 3 cups per day. If using

the seeds, use 1 teaspoon to 1 cup of water, and boil it until the seeds are tender. Eat this like a soup, seeds and all.

## AVAILABILITY
Fenugreek is readily available. It's also easy to grow.

# GOLDENSEAL

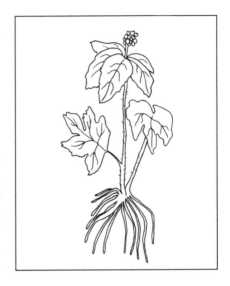

*Hydrastis canadensis*
Also called yellow root, jaundice root, and tumeric

## REPORTED BENEFITS
Jethro Kloss in *Back to Eden* (1988) praises this herb as "one of the most wonderful remedies in the entire herb kingdom . . . a real cure-all." Many North American tribes have used goldenseal extensively, and they taught early American and Canadian settlers how to use it. It was included in the *U.S. Pharmacopoeia* from 1831 to 1936 and considered an astringent; antiseptic; digestion stimulant; tonic to be used during convalescence from colds, fevers, and flu; and aid for eye and skin conditions, sore throat, and complications of childbirth.

Goldenseal has been the chief ingredient in many patent medicines after the U.S. Civil War, notably Dr. Pierce's Golden Medical Discovery. The word *golden* suggests the bright yellow-orange pulp of the root. A century ago you could not purchase the root for less than a dollar a pound (a steep sum in those days), because it was believed to be a tonic that lengthened the life span. It was collected so much in the wild that it became nearly extinct. Today, goldenseal is an important cultivated herb.

This herb, native to North America, has knotty rhizomes of yellowish brown bark and requires 70 percent shade and moisture with good drainage to thrive. It grows from Ontario through New York, to Pennsylvania, West Virginia, Ohio, Kentucky, and Indiana.

Homeopaths have prescribed micro doses for treatment of alcoholism, asthma, indigestion, cancer, hemorrhoids, and liver ailments. Studies show it is a potent antibiotic, good in the treatment of bacterial, fungal, and protozoan infections. It is quite effective for infectious diarrhea caused by such bacteria as salmonella, shigella, and others, as well as protozoans causing amebic dysentery. Several reports have shown it effective against cholera, with one study proving it more powerful and safer than pharmaceutical antibiotics such as Chloromycetin.

It also revs up the immune system, enhancing the production of white blood cells which devour disease-causing microorganisms. Animal experiments have pointed to its ability to shrink tumors, and although no human studies have been done, it may be valuable to those taking chemotherapy.

## TONIC USAGE
Goldenseal is bitter-tasting with a sweet licorice aroma. People with high blood pressure, diabetes, or heart disease should be cautious about using it. In any case, short-term usage is recommended only.

Since the herb is endangered, it is best to gather roots you grow yourself. This can be accomplished if you have plenty of shade or construct shade frames to grow the plants under. Collect only mature, 5-year-old roots. You can count the annual stem scars to determine the plant's age, one for every year. You can also purchase 2-year-old roots from specialty nurseries; so, you won't need to wait so long for harvest. Or simply buy the dried root from a local health food store.

To make a tea, use ½ teaspoon of dried powdered root per cup of water. Bring the tea to a boil, remove from heat, cover, and steep 15 minutes. Drink up to 2 cups per day.

## AVAILABILITY
Growing goldenseal requires a long-term investment and adequate space. Dried root is available in most stores where you purchase dried herbs.

# MULLEIN

*Verbascum thapsus*
Also called hag's taper, donkey's ears, and flannel plant

## REPORTED BENEFITS
This biennial has been naturalized in the United States, Canada, and Australia. Mullein requires full sun and produces a single large flower stalk which looks like a large candle. In fact, it was once made into primitive torches by dipping the stalk in tallow and lighting it. Mullein was not just an herb to light the way in the dark, it was also a glowing medicinal to which Norwegian peasants attributed magical healing qualities. It has been used for lung conditions, coughs, asthma, bronchitis, colds, and tuberculosis. The herb has diuretic properties, checks diarrhea, and reduces inflammation and bleeding bowels. It is mucilaginous and soothes

stomachaches. In Ireland mullein was cultivated extensively for lung treatments. The English have used it for hundreds of years; it is mentioned in nearly every herbal.

It contains potassium and calcium phosphate, two organic salts necessary for the nervous system and bone structure. Research shows that mullein has antiseptic and germicidal qualities, acts as an antispasmodic, calms or quiets nerves, soothes inflamed tissues, and generally promotes rest and sleep.

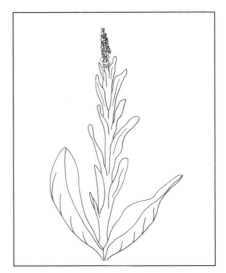

### TONIC USAGE
This herb has been deemed quite safe to take even in large quantities. One study shows no harm even to those consuming over a quart of a brew of this herb a day. Tea made from the flowers is slightly sweet; the leaves are slightly bitter. You can use leaves, flowers, or the root of this plant as you wish. Generally, mullein has been collected from the wild, but a large percentage of the herb available for sale now comes from cultivated plants.

It is best to drink mullein tea in the evening or just before bedtime because of its sleep-inducing property. To make your tea, take ½ cup of fresh leaves, flowers, or both chopped, and pour 1½ pints of boiling water over them. You can substitute ¼ cup of dried leaves and flowers for the fresh, but fresh is best. Cover and steep 15 minutes. You can drink up to 3 cups.

### AVAILABILITY
Mullein may be difficult to purchase, but it's not impossible. Do not disturb wild plants since they are becoming rare. You can grow your own if you find the seed.

# SHEEP SORREL

*Rumex acetosella*
Also called red sorrel and sour weed

### REPORTED BENEFITS
Another herb used in the famous Essiac tonic, sheep sorrel contains oxalic acid, sodium, potassium, iron, manganese, and high amounts of vitamin C, phosphorus, and beta carotene. The plant has snakelike roots which crawl

under the grass sending up small red starts. This little weed has guided farmers through the years regarding soil conditions, because sheep sorrel only grows in the poor soils of fields and open meadows with high acid contents.

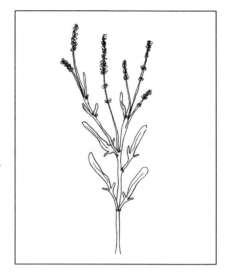

The Latin name means "the little vinegar plant," and sheep sorrel does in fact have a sour taste. The use of the spear-shaped leaves in food can be traced back to ancient Egyptians in 3000 B.C., who enjoyed many dishes made from it. During the reign of Henry VIII of England, it was used as a meat tenderizer, and the leaves were also boiled and eaten like spinach. The English used the mashed leaves with vinegar and sugar to create a green sauce for meats and fish. So, its use as a spring vegetable to spice up tired taste buds ensured that those dining on it also got a dose of vitamins. A traditional Jewish soup, shav, is made with sheep sorrel. In 1895 more than 44 million pounds of sheep sorrel were delivered to markets in France, and it is still popular in French cuisine.

As for being a strengthening herb, sheep sorrel has been used as an ingredient in apothecaries' formulas from the 15th to 19th centuries. They called it herba acetosa. According to 16th century English herbalist John Gerard, "It cooleth the stomache, tempereth the heat of the liver, openeth the stoppings there of." It was often prized as a blood medicine. The herb acts as a diuretic, and research shows it is mildly antiseptic and a light laxative. It was once used to prevent scurvy by virtue of its high vitamin C content. A cooling agent for fevers, sheep sorrel also relieves thirst. According to herbalist James Duke, the leaf tea was considered a folk remedy for cancer. High in many vitamins and minerals, it is an important herb for building up weakened bodies.

## TONIC USAGE

Sheep sorrel has a sharp, sour, slightly lemony taste. An infusion of this is best if chilled and sipped like lemonade. Use the new shoots and leaves when they appear in early spring. Leaves can also be collected through the fall. It is a perennial, native to Europe and Asia, but it has been introduced all over the world, growing wild as a weed. You can propagate the seeds in spring. The plant tolerates partial shade and does well in poor soil. It is rarely seen for sale fresh in the United States and Canada, although more herb shops are beginning to carry the dried form.

Because of its high amount of oxalic acid, people with a tendency toward kidney stones or arthritis should exercise discretion when using this herb.

Use the roots or leaves for medicinal teas. If buying the powdered root, make sure that what you are getting is really sheep sorrel. Some substitutions have been passed off as true sheep sorrel. The powder should be green in color and have the aroma of sweet grass.

For tea, use ½ cup of leaves per pint of boiling water. Let steep 10 minutes and strain. Cool in the refrigerator. Drink 1 to 2 cups per day. For a root decoction, place 1 teaspoon of powdered root into 1 cup of boiling water. Simmer covered 10 minutes, strain, and cool. Drink 1 to 2 cups per day.

## AVAILABILITY
Sheep sorrel is easiest to obtain if you grow it yourself. It may be difficult to obtain a good-quality product dried, and it is almost impossible to buy the herb fresh.

# Energizing Tonic Herbs
## *To Stimulate the Body*

The word *stimulate* suggests a call to action. For the physical body and its health, stimulants can function as a call to life. Stimulants increase metabolism and circulation, often breaking up obstructions and warming the body. They function to jump-start the body into movement, since when something slows down, it eventually stops working. That's not what we want our living machines to do.

Nutrition is key to keeping the body vital. The body's health relies on its absorbing and utilizing proper enzymes, nutrients, and vitamins. If metabolism becomes sluggish, the body cannot properly assimilate these things. That's why it is so important to stimulate the system when it seems bogged down. As the body speeds up, new cells are created, and these new cells can in turn utilize the necessary nutrition.

Certain types of herbs act as stimulants to speed up sluggish metabolism. These herbs contain specific vitamins, minerals, and enzymes which help prevent oxidation damage to cell membranes caused by free radicals (atoms that cause cell damage, created by toxins, wastes, and imbalances within the body). Scientists claim oxidation damage is one of the main mechanisms causing aging. A group of vitamins called antioxidants act as free-radical scavengers, eating up these little devils and protecting the body from degenerative diseases by invigorating cell life. Stimulating herbs contain perhaps the highest amounts of these antioxidants that act not only as energizers for the body but also as a type of super fuel to keep it running at tip-top efficiency and health.

These stimulants should be avoided by pregnant women and people with especially weak health. Use the stimulant 2 to 3 weeks, allow the body to rest 1 week, and resume as necessary.

## CAYENNE

*Capsicum annuum*

### REPORTED BENEFITS
South American tribes enjoyed hot pepper meals as far back as 500 B.C. It is popular in the cuisines of India, China, South Africa, and Mexico. This pepper is native to subtropical America, but cayenne has been grown as an annual in gardens all over the world. And yet, we would never imagine that

this hot spice would be valuable as a medicinal. It is one of the most useful and popular stimulants in the herb world. Herbalists all agree that cayenne cannot be beat as an energy stimulant. Herbalist Jethro Kloss has called it one of "the most wonderful herb medicines we have." And herbalist R. C. Wren claims it is "the purest and most certain stimulant in herbal materia medica . . ."

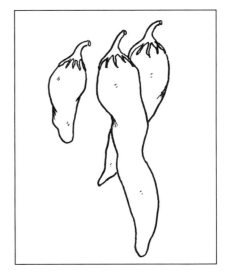

No wonder cayenne has earned such praises, for it has many health claims. For one, cayenne encourages the adrenal glands to produce a light amount of cortisone. This makes it a wonder for skin problems. One clinical study demonstrated that 75 percent of the people who applied a cream made of cayenne to shingles experienced substantial pain relief. The action of this herb brings blood and body heat to the surface, stimulates sweating and hence cooling the body, stabilizes blood pressure, and reduces excess bleeding. West Indians often soaked the pods in hot water, added sugar and sour orange juice, and drank it freely to rid themselves of fevers.

Not only that, but dieters should take notice, since cayenne temporarily boosts the body's metabolic rate 25 percent, speeding up its ability to burn off extra calories. Researchers at Oxford Polytechnic in England found that cayenne burned up those extra calories faster than other foods. Since it is a powerful stimulant that's often used as a hangover treatment, cayenne, as you probably guessed, is also vitamin-packed. It contains large amounts of vitamin C, A (a whopping 21,600 IU per 3½ ounces), iron, potassium, and niacin.

Cayenne is wonderful for reducing sinus congestion and ridding the body of colds, because it contains antiseptic qualities. The Hunan and Szechwan people in China who steep meals in hot peppers have been found to have less chronic obstructive lung disease than people in China with blander diets. Many herbalists have agreed that cold symptoms can be eliminated with only 1 to 2 doses of cayenne powder taken in warm water.

## TONIC USAGE

If you do any gardening at all, it is easy to plant three or four cayenne plants at the edge of your garden or patio, which could easily provide you with all the hot peppers or powder to last a year. The plants grow 2 feet high and

85

need 14- to 18-week growing periods. Harvest the fruit pods when they turn bright red. Be careful not to rub your eyes after handling and wear gloves whenever touching them. You can dry the pods easily by threading them together on a string and hanging them in the kitchen for 3 to 4 weeks. After they have dried completely you can make a fine powder by grinding them in a food processor. Just make sure you don't inhale the dust, or you'll be sorry. Pour the powder into a lidded jar and label it, keeping it in a cool, dry place until you are ready to use it.

To use, add ½ teaspoon to a ½ cup of boiling water, stir, and let the water cool to room temperature. You may wish to add other herbs to the tea if you don't like spicy foods. Just be sure not to drink over 1 cup, since large doses can irritate the gastrointestinal system.

## AVAILABILITY
Cayenne is readily available in grocery or health food stores. You can even purchase it through the mail from spice companies. You can also buy hot peppers at produce stands in season.

# EVENING PRIMROSE

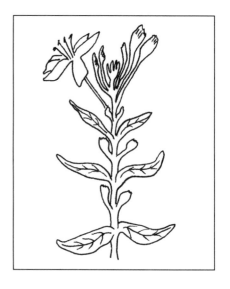

*Oenothera biennis*
Also called evening star and cure-all

## REPORTED BENEFITS
Evening primrose oil recently received attention from pharmaceutical companies because it was discovered to contain a compound that reduces the rate of blood clotting, which helps prevent some forms of heart attack. Many other claims have been made for this herb. Perhaps that is why it is such a showy plant, which blooms at night all summer. Evening primrose is easy to grow, it's also native to North America; the plant self-sows and gets by with little attention. That's a good thing, since it has been neglected in the past in herbal medicine.

Although ancient Greeks ate the roots to promote their appetite for wine, and Germans still eat them as an aperitif, it really wasn't until the 1980s that evening primrose achieved any real medical acclaim. The main discovery was that it contains gamma-linoleic acid that's helpful in preventing heart attacks, reducing high blood pressure, guarding against coronary artery disease, and keeping hair and nails healthy. All parts of the plant are edible and nutritious. The plant soothes and protects mucous membranes, acts as an antispasmodic, and serves as a weak astringent.

In a 1981 clinical study at St. Thomas Hospital in London, 61 percent of subjects with premenstrual syndrome who took evening primrose found that symptoms disappeared, while 23 percent found partial relief. In another 1981 study in Scotland at Glasgow Royal Infirmary, 60 percent of patients found improvement of rheumatoid arthritis while taking the evening primrose oil and fish oil instead of regular drugs. The most potent source of gamma-linoleic acid from the plant is contained in the seeds, and it strengthens the body by suppressing substances in the body causing inflammation. But it does not suppress the immune system. For people on conventional rheumatoid arthritis treatments, which weaken the immune system, this is wonderful. A 1993 study at the University of Pennsylvania and the University of Massachusetts reported significant decreases in joint pain, tenderness, and swelling when sufferers were given capsules containing gamma-linoleic acid.

Another Scottish study, done by Highland Psychiatric Research Group, found that evening primrose encouraged regeneration of liver cells damaged in alcoholism. Researchers also believe it may prevent alcohol poisoning, hangovers, post-drinking depression, alcohol-withdrawal symptoms, and it may even prevent brain damage to cells from alcohol. But more studies need to be done for conclusive evidence. We do know that evening primrose helps headaches and depression; so, if the herb does help an alcohol-ravaged body it will indeed prove to be a powerful stimulant.

## TONIC USAGE
You can use all parts of the evening primrose plant: the leaves and flowers, the root, and the seed. Perhaps it's easiest to use the leaves and flowers. To make your tonic, boil 2 cups of water. Remove from heat, and add ½ cup of fresh leaves and flowers or ¼ cup of dried leaves and flowers. Let the tea stand covered for 15 minutes, then strain, and drink throughout the day or in the evening.

## AVAILABILITY
Evening primrose essential oil is available at health food stores. For plant material, you may wish to grow your own if you have enough space. The flowers glow beautifully at night with a heavenly scent.

# GINKGO

*Ginkgo biloba*
Also called maidenhair tree

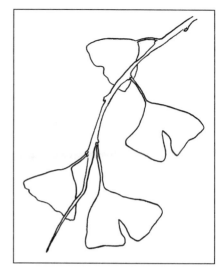

## REPORTED BENEFITS

This healing tree, with male and female species, is very ornamental and blooms in the summer. Ginkgo is one of the oldest living tree species, dating to the Permian period (230 million years ago) of the Paleozoic era. But it no longer grows wild, and perhaps the only reason we have it today is that Chinese monks, who thought of the tree as sacred, cultivated it for centuries. Otherwise, it would likely have disappeared into the mists of time. The Japanese word *ginkyo* means "silver apricot," and although the ginkgo produces a smelly fruit, it is prized in Japanese and Chinese restaurants as a delicacy. Some suppose the smell, slightly reminiscent of vomit, was a protection against dinosaurs. Cooking and adding sweetener makes the fruit quite palatable; it is unpleasant only in its raw state. The cooked nut within the fruit can also be eaten.

Ginkgo is rapidly gaining recognition as a brain tonic that enhances memory. It increases blood flow and metabolism efficiency, regulates neurotransmitters, and boosts oxygen levels in the brain. A study involving healthy young women showed that memory was dramatically increased after a large dose of the extract was given. Studies are now being conducted on its use in Alzheimer's disease. It also helps reduce hearing loss and circulation-related disorders like diabetes and phlebitis. Ginkgo also reportedly helps people with asthma. In one study, asthmatic children found relief while taking an extract. The leaves can help lift depression, increase blood flow, reduce kidney disorders, stimulate the immune system, discourage formation of arterial plaque, prevent toxic shock syndrome, reduce edema, and diminish the effects of alcohol. The herb destroys free radicals and may even help prevent cancer.

## TONIC USAGE

The ginkgo tree is closely related to conifers, but it has broad, fan-shaped leaves. It is a strange, hardy tree, and if you dare to gather the fruit, wear disposable gloves, since the smell can transfer onto the skin.

For use as a tonic, you don't have to bother with the fruit; simply use the leaves to make a tincture. Wait until the leaves turn yellow in fall. Fill a jar with the leaves and cover it with vodka. Seal and let it stand 2 weeks. Strain and store in a dark, cool place. To make your tea, place 1 tablespoon of leaves in 1 cup of boiling water, cover, and let cool 15 minutes. Virtually all the alcohol will evaporate due to the hot water; so, this is an excellent way to obtain a good concentrate of plant material.

## AVAILABILITY
Since the ginkgo tree is rare but easy to grow, you can purchase it through some specialty nurseries. It makes a fun addition to the landscape. However, the ginkgo extract can be found in health food stores.

# MINT

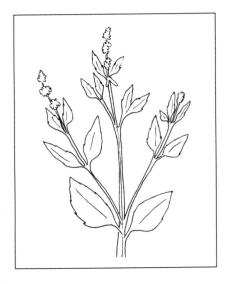

*Mentha x piperita*
Also called peppermint and lamb mint

## REPORTED BENEFITS
Mint is a common herb used in flavorings and candy. Originally there were 25 true species of mint from Europe and Asia, but mints have been hybridized extensively. Peppermint is generally thought to be richest in essential oils and the most active in stimulant properties of all the mints. Just like evening primrose, mint is a newcomer to herbal medicines. English botanist John Ray mentioned it in 1696 in one of his papers. In 1721, mint was listed in the *London Pharmacopeia* as a digestive aid and flavoring.

Peppermint is an effective and instantaneous cure for nausea, as well as a tasty tea which soothes most stomach upsets. Since it contains menthol, azulene, vitamins C and E, and bioflavonoids, it packs quite a nutritive punch. Peppermint also contains phenolic-type antioxidants in abundance. It increases stomach acidity, which is essential for digestion, and relaxes muscles in the digestive tract. The bioflavonoids stimulate the gallbladder to contract and secrete bile. If the tea is drunk before eating, hunger pangs will disappear, then return later with stronger force; so, in effect, peppermint increases appetite. Studies show it relieves colon spasms and is found to be a specific remedy for irritable bowel syndrome. It also decreases inflammation; so, it is useful for gout and ulcers. It also helps reduce headaches and migraines, kills bacteria and viruses in the stomach, and balances the intestinal flora. The herb can also aid in calming the nerves. This gentle stimulant has been given to children to stop them from vomiting. It is useful for debility since it fortifies the organs, rallies strength, and serves as a stimulant.

Dioscorides claimed mint was an aphrodisiac, which essentially means it was considered a stimulant. The *U.S. Dispensatory* notes that peppermint "is generally regarded as an excellent carminative and gastric stimulant . . ." Today, it is probably the most extensively used herb in the world, with thousands of acres cultivated to meet the demand. Who hasn't taken a cup of peppermint tea to bed to soothe a tummy ache? Perhaps we should drink it more often. As part of a tonic program, peppermint is important not only by itself, but as a flavoring to make more bitter brews easier to swallow.

## TONIC USAGE
This herb is good in a tonic tea, hot or cold. Mint is an easy-to-grow perennial which spreads easily and likes sun. It is easily propagated through root division. The tea has a strong mint taste, fresh and clean.

Gather the leaves and flower tips just after it has bloomed. Dry by laying it out on newspapers in a dark place for 4 to 5 days. Crumble lightly and place the mint in a tightly closed jar. Make your tea by adding 1 teaspoon of dried or 3 teaspoons of fresh mint to 1 cup of boiling water. Steep 10 minutes covered, strain, and drink. Drink up to 3 cups per day.

## AVAILABILITY
Mint is readily available; you can even find peppermint tea at regular grocery stores. If you grow the herb, beware, since it tends to take over wherever it is planted.


# PARSLEY

*Petroselinum crispum*
Also called carum

## REPORTED BENEFITS
Parsley is a so-called sweet herb because it is so rich in chlorophyll that it even removes garlic and onion odors on the breath. This use is still popular today. Garlands of parsley were worn at ancient Greek and Roman banquets with the notion that the herb prevented intoxication. An old prescription from Hippocrates' temple on the Greek island of Cos contained parsley, as

well as herbs like thyme, fennel, and anise, powdered and mixed with wine. This mixture is thought to be the basis for many tonics and cure-alls in the Middle Ages.

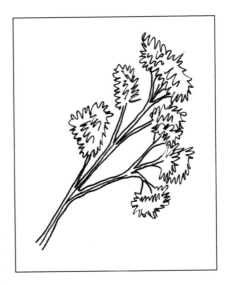

Herbalists today value parsley for its use in helping arthritis and rheumatism. It also is good for asthma, coughs, and urinary disorders, since it contains a rich abundance of vitamins A, B, C, and K, as well as iron, iodine, phosphorus, potassium, and calcium. It inhibits histamine and so reduces inflammation, and it is important as a free-radical scavenger. Studies show that parsley contains a substance in which tumor cells cannot multiply. Physicians in the United States and Canada continue to prescribe the tea to young women with bladder problems. The herb is good for liver and kidney function. Today the essential oil is used in some pharmaceuticals for kidney ailments and to induce menstruation. For centuries, the root has been considered a stimulant and a laxative, good for obesity, edema, fluid retention, and excessive gas.

## TONIC USAGE
This biennial is a member of the carrot family, and its rich tea flavor is at once refreshing and cooling. Parsley can take partial shade and is easy to grow.

To make parsley tea, harvest the leaves and stems right before the plant flowers. Or if you wish, dig up the roots and dry them in a low oven, powdering them in a food processor. Add 1 teaspoon of fresh leaves or 3 teaspoons of dried leaves to 1 cup of boiling water, cover, and steep 15 to 20 minutes. Then strain and drink up to 2 cups per day. For the powdered root, use ½ teaspoon in 1 cup of boiling water, simmer covered 10 minutes, strain, and drink 1 cup per day. It should be noted that the essential oil should only be used under medical supervision. Large intake can cause abortions and irritate internal organs; so use care.

## AVAILABILITY
Parsley is available commercially in fresh-leaf and dried forms. Sometimes the root can be found, but this is rare. The herb is easy to grow in the garden or as a border for a flower bed.

# ROSE HIPS

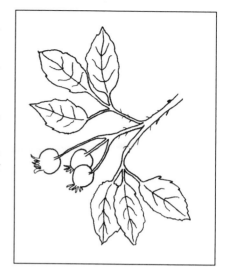

*Rosa rugosa*
Also called fruit from the rugosa rose

## REPORTED BENEFITS

If you had to, you could make your own vitamins with rose hips. Rose hips, taken from the fruit of the rugosa rose, have a richer abundance of vitamin C than orange juice, ounce-for-ounce. Just a tiny handful of these round wonders can provide vitamin C that's the value of 60 oranges! Rose hips also contain vitamins A, $B_1$, and $B_2$, as well as pectin and zinc. They are considered a tonic with laxative and astringent properties. They have been used to banish lethargy. With large quantities of antioxidant vitamin C, rose hips make a powerful yet safe stimulant.

During World War II, rose hips were the sole source of vitamin C in some areas, and this rose fruit has been credited for the general good health of many people during that war. In Norway and Sweden, wild hips are still collected from fields or at the edges of woodlands to add to soups or stews or to make into preserves and juices to fortify what could be a vitamin-poor winter menu. The *British Phamacopoeia* lists only *Rosa galica*, but most old roses are medicinal, and the *rugosa* has the largest hips. Many herbalists have suggested that rose-hip tea should be part of a daily diet.

## TONIC USAGE

With its tart, cranberrylike taste—spicy and fruity—and so much going for it, it's hard to believe that rose hips are free for the taking in fall, after roses have finished blooming for the season. It is not difficult to grow roses in the yard, since you can enjoy the blooms all summer and the hips all winter. The *hip* is the ripened accessory fruit of a rose that consists of a fleshy receptacle that encloses numerous achenes.

Gather the round "berries," or hips, appearing on the rosebush just when they turn bright scarlet (not dark red; then they're overripe). Usually the hips ripen just after the first frost. Roses grown in colder latitudes produce rose hips with the highest concentrations of vitamin C. Perhaps this is nature's way of taking care of people who have to endure bitter weather. After collecting the hips, wash and trim the blossom and stem ends; then chill them immediately. You can seal rose hips in a plastic bag and freeze them up to

6 months. Chilling is necessary to inactivate enzymes which might cause vitamin loss, if you plan to prepare them for use within the next day or so.

Care must be taken in preparation of your tonic. Avoid using copper or aluminum pans to make your tea since these metals affect the vitamin content. It's best to use glass or enamel pans with wooden spoons. To make your tincture, use 1 cup of hips and 1½ cups of water, heat to boiling, then cover, reduce heat, and simmer 15 minutes. Next, let it stand for 24 hours. Strain this mixture and bring it again to a rolling boil, adding 2 tablespoons of lemon juice for each pint. Store the tincture in the refrigerator, adding honey for taste. You can then add 2 tablespoons of this tincture to your morning juice or to 1 cup of warm water for a tea.

## AVAILABILITY
Rose hips are readily available. You can purchase rosebushes at most nurseries. Rose hips can also be purchased at health food and herb shops.

# SASSAFRAS

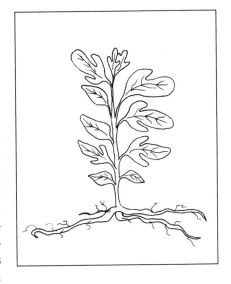

*Sassafras albidum*
Also called ague tree and cinnamon wood

## REPORTED BENEFITS
Sassafras is another tree that acts as a stimulant and that has been used as a spring tonic or blood purifier for quite some time. A member of the laurel family, sassafras is native to the North American woods and was used by native tribes long before European settlers arrived. North American tribes used the bark soaked in water as an antiseptic wash for wounds and for the eyes. News about sassafras spread quickly. In 1569 Monardes, a Spanish physician, wrote that this medicinal also made a tasty tea.

Herbalists agree that sassafras helps gout and arthritis, can be useful in inducing perspiration and urination, and reduces fevers. It also has stimulant and antiseptic properties. When you drink sassafras tea, the herb creates a warming sensation. It improves digestion and reduces high blood pressure. For thousands of years, people have drunk and used this reddish brown fragrant tea with no ill effects. Sassafras was once a popular flavoring and ingredient in the original root beer, as well as an ingredient in many patent medicines.

Herbalist Dr. Edward E. Shook recommended use of the yellowish liquid from recently fallen trees, which contained only small concentrations of safrole, thought to be dangerous. He cautioned that if taken in large quantity or over extended periods of time, sassafras can be poisonous. The physician quoted an old saying, "It takes a poison to kill a poison." This may be true in the case of sassafras, and this is indeed the backbone of homeopathic medicine and of vaccines. Sassafras is still recognized in Ozark folk medicine; a 1734 recipe for a cancer remedy states that sassafras "should be drunk every morning . . . along with moderate living." This stimulant has been used to treat everything, even syphilis, along with sarsaparilla.

## TONIC USAGE

Sassafras tree stems are covered in rough, reddish brown bark that attracts the tiger swallowtail butterfly. It grows in sun or partial shade and has alternate leaves appearing in three forms. One leaf is simple, another is mittenlike, and a third is three-lobed.

The U.S. Food & Drug Administration (FDA) has banned the use of sassafras for consumption. Historically, the tonic was made from the root, which is as thick as an arm or thigh, gray outside and red inside, and very sweet-smelling. However, the leaves have also been used, and have small concentrations of safrole. A tea was made by taking 1 teaspoon of shaved root bark added to 1 cup of water and brought to a boil. The heat was reduced, the pot covered, and left to simmer for 20 minutes. After straining, the tea was drunk 1 cup per day for 2 to 3 days. The tea was also good cold.

Exercise caution with this herb.

## AVAILABILITY

Sassafras is not readily available. Trees can be purchased for ornamental growth.


# STINGING NETTLE

*Urtica dioica*
Also called Indian spinach and hokey-pokey

## REPORTED BENEFITS

The leaves of this bushy weed contain hairs which sting like bees and inject stinging venom into the skin in much the same way. Researchers have discovered that the hairs contain formic acid, histamine, and acetylcholine, which together create burning, then itching. Perhaps the plant is merely trying to protect the potent healing juices within. In the 10th century stinging nettle was listed as one of the nine powerful herbs which combatted "evils." According to English herbalist John Gerard, it was a poison antidote.

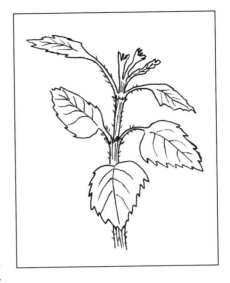

Traditionally a spring tonic, stinging nettle was taken to stimulate the kidneys, rid the body of worms, cure diarrhea, help asthma, stop internal bleeding, and purify the blood. Both the seeds and flowers were once used in a wine-based tonic to combat fevers. The seeds have also been used to treat everything from bat bites to heavy-metal toxicity. Swiss naturalist Conrad Gesner (1516–1565) recommended the root for jaundice. Stinging nettle stimulates the digestive system, acts as an astringent, and helps reduce cold symptoms. It also aids the liver and lungs and is good for pleurisy. The herb is diuretic, and the tea has been sipped to relieve arthritis and gout. Amazingly, stinging nettle is a pain reliever that's also good for anemia, poor circulation, and lowering blood sugar. Australian aborigines used a nettle lotion for sprains and boiled the leaves to make poultices. And studies at the University of Lund in Sweden revealed that water containing dried or fresh nettle poured on plants stimulated their growth, proving that the herb is a rich, nutritive addition to the diet, whether plant or human.

Nettle is "rich in easily digested and assimilated protein, minerals, vitamins, micronutrients," says Susun Weed in *Healing Wise* (1989). "It rebuilds the kidneys (seat of chi) and adrenals (seat of energy). It nourishes energy in nerves, the immune system, and the circulatory system. It enhances mental clarity and physical endurance. Nettle is an ally which . . . can help the gradual healing of a person with a chronic condition such as Epstein-Barr virus (EBV), hay fever, allergies, lymphatic swellings, ARC/AIDS, nerve inflammations (including lumbago and sciatica), persistent headaches, high blood pressure, inexplicable lethargy and exhaustion, repeated bouts of flu and colds, hardened arteries, weakened veins, infertility, rheumatism, joint aches, continuous skin eruptions, and loss of nerve sensitivity. . . . Nettle infusions heal kidney cells like nothing else I've ever seen." It contains high amounts of vitamins C, D, A, and K, and is rich in iron (and vitamin C aids in iron absorption), protein, potassium, magnesium, iodine, chlorophyll, and formic acid.

## TONIC USAGE

Archaeologists have actually found nettle fabric wrapped around a body in a Bronze Age burial site in Denmark. And during the cotton shortage of World War I, Germans substituted nettle. It can be found all over the world around waste dumps and roadsides. With its "stinging," one would suppose that such an herb, instead of being protective and healing, would actually be harmful. But herbalists use only the young shoots and leaves in early spring which do not yet contain the stinging hairs.

The tea has a bland green taste; it's brothlike. To gather nettle, use gloves for protection and take only young leaves. Dry them out on newspapers in a dark place for several days, then crumble them, and place them in a tightly closed jar. Use 2 teaspoons added to 1 cup of boiling water, cover, and let steep 5 to 10 minutes. Drink 1 to 2 cups per day. You can also add the leaves to salads and eat them steamed like spinach.

You can easily establish a bed of nettle, perhaps in some out-of-the-way corner of your yard. But beware. Once established, they spread easily with their creeping rootstocks. Nettle is rarely cultivated, but when it is, it's for medicinal purposes.

## AVAILABILITY

Nettle is very common along riverbanks and wild places, but be sure to know what it is you're gathering. Seed can sometimes be purchased and may be found in dried form from a few herb companies.

# VIOLET

*Viola papilionacea*
Also called wild violet

## REPORTED BENEFITS

Violet, a mild stimulant, was a symbol of ancient fertility, depicted in love scenes in medieval tapestries. It is also a delightful spring plant with tiny blue flowers and deep green, heart-shaped leaves. It spreads rapidly, likes partial shade, and grows wild in meadows and along the edges of trails and paths.

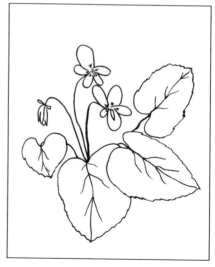

Contained within the leaves and flowers are rutin (which strengthens capillaries), vitamin C, and vitamin A. It is a traditional folk treatment for cancer, especially breast cancer, taken either internally or used as a poultice. Its cancer-healing claims (by simple ingestion of an infusion) have drawn contemporary interest. Experiments in 1960 showed the extract inhibited tumors on mice. It also contains an aspirinlike substance, relieves sinus congestion, and helps clear lungs of respiratory disorders. It's helpful for arthritis and infections. Since it has a cooling nature, herbalists like to use it in cough mixtures. It has been hailed as a blood purifier. Violet also relieves anxiety and insomnia, acts as a gentle laxative, and lowers high blood pressure. Studies done in Pakistan show that it increases sweating, reduces fevers, and relieves headaches.

## TONIC USAGE
Only the odorless wild American violet, of the over 200 different species of violet, is used medicinally. The European sweet violet is used in perfumery.

The tonic tea produces a mild, sweet, slightly peppery drink with a mucilaginous—slightly gummy—texture. Collect and dry the flowers and leaves in early spring. In the past, violet flowers were candied and made into jams. Dry leaves and flowers on newspapers in a dark area for several days until crumbly. Store in a tightly closed jar. Add 1 teaspoon of dried violet or 3 teaspoons of fresh violet to 1 cup of boiling water. Cover and steep 10 minutes. Drink up to 3 cups per day.

## AVAILABILITY
Violet may be hard to purchase dried. Check wildflower catalogs to purchase plants or seed. You will soon have a patch to harvest year after year, without any bother.

# Renewing Tonic Herbs
### To Ease Stress, Tension, and Depression

Our daily lives are filled with change, and with change often comes stress. We worry about finances, social obligations, health, family, friends, or jobs. Friends and lovers come and go. We live with surprises and disappointments. Usually, our bodies manage to adjust to these changes and this stress. But when many changes arrive all at once and cause serious alterations in our lives, or if we don't take care of the body properly, that's when usually dependable body functions break down.

When the body is overwhelmed or "overstressed," this may lead to depression. Although depression begins in the limbic part of the brain, which affects mood, it can also affect us physically. Tension tightens the shoulders, and sadness weighs heavily on facial features. We experience loss or increase in appetite. Perhaps we experience headaches, backaches, digestion difficulties, or feelings of worthlessness or inadequacy. Our energy level drops. We find ourselves coping with insomnia or sleeping too much. Dr. John A. Schindler in *How to Live 365 Days a Year* (1975) asserts that 35 to 50 percent of people are sick because they are unhappy. That's an eye-opening statistic, but one we intuitively know is true. How many of us have experienced stress overload? Or, how many of us have not had at least one bout with depression? And what usually happens when we are going through such emotional upsets? If we pay close attention, we realize that we usually end up with a cold, flu, or a more dangerous illness.

"Digestion is important to relaxation and the body's ability to handle an overload of stress. And then again, relaxation is key to digestion. It *is* a circle," herbalist Harriet Prosperi says. "If you eat when you are upset or angry, excited, or under severe stress, you will have indigestion. Our bodies simply will be unable to use the nutrients from the food we have eaten. If digestion is incomplete, you are short-changing your body. Adrenal function will become impaired. The adrenal glands, located on top of each kidney, are responsible for the maintenance of salt and water balance in the body, and also the production of certain hormones, most importantly, adrenaline, which is the hormone needed in our bodies' response to stress."

So, how do we stop this merry-go-round? Ohio herbalist and lecturer Rae Jean Elliott adds, "There are herbs you can choose to use which have a calming effect on the nervous system, allowing for the release of tension and stress, and also for working on the digestive system. Stress does directly affect the digestive process and, in turn, adrenal functioning. And this is what leads to other physical problems. The herbs can relieve all these symptoms, and the best news of all, they aren't addictive or habit-forming either."

By using certain herbs, we can stop this endless cycle. Specific herbs that relax us and reestablish our natural balance are useful for boosting blood and nourishment to the brain, combating depression, and supporting the body's adrenal function so that the mechanism which helps the body deal with stress can again work smoothly.

Whenever you begin to feel you're under stress, depressed, or tense, don't waste a moment. Attend to this state of your body, whatever the cause—poor nutritional habits, not enough exercise, or just too much activity in your life. Take positive action to relieve the stress, and prepare a renewing tonic herb that best suits your situation.

The fourteen tonic herbs described in this chapter may be used to relax and relieve stress in your life. However, since most are sedative, the best time to take them is at bedtime. If you do take them during the day, make sure you do not drive or operate machinery. Use these herbs only as necessary until symptoms are gone—up to one week only. If needed, rest 3 days and resume taking the herb for another week.

Renewing tonic herbs all share an ability to act as a sedative and as a stimulant in some way. Although you should exercise caution with dosage, many of these herbs do not have the nasty side effects of many manufactured drugs because these herbs work in the body in a natural way.

# BARBERRY

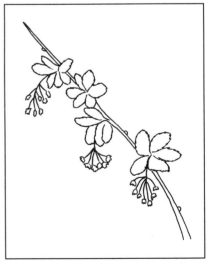

*Berberis vulgaris*
Also called sowberry and jaundice berry

### REPORTED BENEFITS
Barberry is an interesting example of how an herb can help specifically in one way, and yet have other healing attributes which work together for the good of the whole body. Like most renewing tonic herbs, it acts both as a sedative and a stimulant.

In ancient Egypt, barberry was made into a syrup mixed with fennel seed to prevent plague. In Europe during the Middle Ages, it was prescribed as a tonic, purgative, and antiseptic. In North America, native tribes prepared decoctions from its root bark to improve appetite and to restore the body from fatigue. It had a wide range of uses from its ability to help soothe a sore throat to controlling diarrhea, relieving jaundice, and cleansing the liver and spleen. Laboratory studies indicate that barberry has stimulant effects on the heart in low doses and depressant effects in high doses. So, caution is advised. But it does contain berberine, which has sedative, anticonvulsant, and stimulant properties (especially for the uterus).

But barberry is rapidly becoming scarce. Long ago farmers called it a blight plant, responsible for ruining their wheat crops, and they destroyed barberry wherever they found it. Later, it was discovered that barberry is a host plant for wheat rust. Now we understand that barberry was not the cause at all. Herbalists relate barberry to Oregon grape, except that barberry contains slightly higher concentrations of berberine and can be used more specifically for the stomach and digestive organs. It stimulates intestinal movements, decreases heart rate, and reduces bronchial constriction.

This perennial shrub grows easily in the sun. Deciduous or evergreen varieties are available, and the purplish fruit develops in late summer or fall. Either the root bark or the berries can be used. The berries, containing high concentrations of vitamin C, can be made into a juice that tastes a little like lemonade when mixed with honey. It's good for scurvy and dysentery. Concentrated juice from the berries is used today in preparing tablets for firming teeth and gums. The berries can also be substituted for cranberries or rose hips in recipes.

## TONIC USAGE
You can obtain barberry from seed or cuttings. A dwarf variety, hardy throughout most of the United States and southern Canada, grows 2 to 5 feet. The common variety grows 4 to 8 feet. The round fruits or berries develop in late summer or fall. To make a tonic tea, use fresh berries (or prepare a syrup with them the same way as for rose hips), taking 1 tablespoon of berries in a cup and covering with boiling water. Cover and steep 15 minutes. Strain. The root bark tonic tea is a bitter and perhaps a stronger sedative. Take 2 tablespoons of fresh root bark, or 1 tablespoon of dried and powdered root bark, and add it to 1 pint of water. Bring to a boil, cover, and reduce heat to a simmer for 15 minutes. Strain. You can drink 1 to 2 cups at bedtime or whenever you feel especially under stress.

## AVAILABILITY
Barberry may be hard to obtain fresh or dried. You can purchase plants at some nurseries.

# BASIL

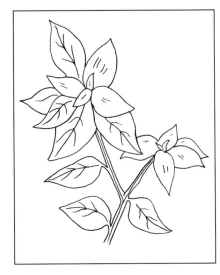

**Ocimum basilicum**
Also called sweet basil and common
basil

## REPORTED BENEFITS

Down through the ages, many herbalists have praised basil. The Greek
physician and botanist Chrysippos de-
clared it his favorite in 400 B.C. And,
in fact, basil means "royal," and roy-
als through the centuries have enjoyed food flavored with it. Today this
popular culinary herb, often used in
tomato dishes, is not thought of as medicinal. Yet it has many health benefits.

There are over 150 different species of basil. Native to India, basil has been
cultivated in the Mediterranean for thousands of years. Holy basil (*Ocimum
sanctum*) is used in Hindu religious ceremonies. Studies of patients at King
George Medical College in India found that this particular species prevents
peptic ulcers and other stress-related diseases, like hypertension, colitis, and
asthma. The leaves of all species of basil help with indigestion and nausea,
and act as gentle sedatives. They are also good for relieving joint pain and
congestion, and they reduce fever in colds and flu. Dried basil was often
provided to 16th century sufferers as a snuff for headaches and head colds.
According to John Gerard in *Gerard's Herbal* (1597), "The smell of basil is
good for the heart . . . It taketh away . . . melancholy . . ."

Aromatherapists use massage oils made with the essential oil of this herb
to decrease mental fatigue and clear the head. Its weak sedative action has
also been used by herbalists to treat anxiety, headaches, and many stomach
and intestinal complaints. Its sedative action contrasts with certain stimulant
properties, allowing it to calm the body from anxiety but stimulate appetite.
Gilbert advised its use in atonic neurosis. Herbalists have often recommended this member of the mint family as an after-dinner aid for digestion
and expelling gas. Clinical studies show that extracts from the seeds dem-
onstrate antibacterial action. It is considered a tonic for the digestive system.

## TONIC USAGE

Basil is a pretty annual that grows 18 inches tall and has a spicy scent. It
grows easily from seed. To harvest for tonic usage, cut the leaves just before
the plant blooms in midsummer. You'll want to use it fresh. Use 1 teaspoon

per cup of boiling water, cover, and let steep 10 to 15 minutes, then strain. Drink up to 3 cups per day. Gather seeds in the fall, adding ½ teaspoon to 1 cup of boiling water, reduce heat, simmer 15 minutes, and strain. The seeds, if kept moisture-free, can be stored in a tightly closed jar for winter use. In winter, you can stuff a handful of leaves into a 1-quart Mason jar. Cover it with vodka, close tightly, and set in a sunny window 1 to 2 weeks. Repeat, replacing old plant material and adding fresh until there is a strong scent which will result in a strong tincture. Add ½ teaspoon of this vodka and basil tincture to a cup of boiling water, adding lemon if you wish. Let cool until room temperature, and stir well.

## AVAILABILITY
Basil is commercially grown in France, Hungary, Bulgaria, Yugoslavia, Italy, and Morocco. It is widely available in grocery stores since it is used as a culinary herb. Seeds can be purchased through any seed catalog.

# BETONY

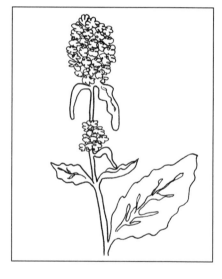

*Stachys officinalis*
Also called wood betony and wound-wort

## REPORTED BENEFITS
"If only we could have as many virtues as betony" is an old Spanish saying. Betony was so useful to ancient Egyptians that they regarded it as magical. Even woodland animals seek this plant out when they are sick or wounded; that tells you something. The Romans listed betony in a treatise written by Antonius Musa, claiming that the herb could cure up to 47 different illnesses. In the latter half of the 17th century, over 30 medicinal uses were recorded. And herbalists still value it, although modern medicine only recognizes its astringent properties.

Herbalist John Lust in *The Herb Book* (1983) lists medicinal uses like help for asthma, bronchitis, heartburn, and kidney problems. Betony has been considered good for throat irritations and diarrhea. The French have recommended the leaves for lung, liver, and gallbladder problems. It contains a phytochemical called trigonelline that's also contained in fenugreek and that has been shown to lower blood-sugar levels.

As for its ability to renew the body under stress, scientists in the Soviet Union found it contains a mixture of glycosides, which are somewhat effective in lowering blood pressure. Betony has been used for headaches and mild anxiety attacks. Sir William Hookers, original director of the Royal Botanical Gardens in Kew, Surrey, claims the name *betony* is a corruption of Celtic words for "head tonic," and it is believed to help ease nervous tension and to act as a natural painkiller. The *Medicina Britannica* (1666) states, "I have known obstinate headaches cured . . . on a decoction of betony."

## TONIC USAGE
A hardy perennial with reddish purple blooms in late summer, betony enjoys full sun or partial shade. It has a musky odor and is self-seeding. It does grow wild. To make your tea, use the leaves, which taste slightly bitter but pleasant and warm. Add 1 teaspoon of dried or 3 teaspoons of fresh leaves to 1 cup of boiling water. Cover and steep 10 to 15 minutes. Strain and add honey if you wish. Drink no more than 2 cups per day, preferably at bedtime.

## AVAILABILITY
Betony can be purchased at herb and health food shops. It is easy to grow.

# BLACK COHOSH

*Cimicifuga racemosa*
Also called squaw root and rattle weed

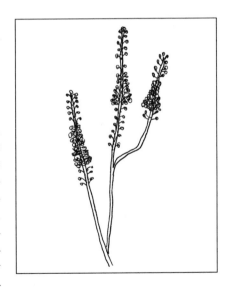

## REPORTED BENEFITS
Black cohosh has traditionally been called a woman's herb, since it acts specifically on the uterus. It causes the uterus to contract, increases menstrual flow, and relieves pain, morning sickness, and menstrual cramps. Both a uterine stimulant and a relaxant, black cohosh possesses estrogen-like qualities. It is unique in its ability to stimulate contractions while relaxing the tension and stress concentrated in uterine muscles.

Although it is an alterative herb (like herbs described in the next chapter), black cohosh also has relaxant qualities which make it a nervine tonic

103

that, as herbalist Dr. Edward Shook declares in *Advanced Treatise in Herbology* (1993), is "one of the most valuable and versatile remedies." Dr. O. Phelps Brown, famed English herbalist, has stated that the root is valuable for inflammation of the nerves, old ulcers, rheumatism, and is also a superior tonic remedy for a variety of chronic diseases. It has diuretic, expectorant, and antispasmodic properties as well as being a sedative. Black cohosh is a bitter and mild expectorant. It depresses the pulse rate but increases the force of the pulse. The Chinese, who call it *sheng ma*, use the herb for treatment in headaches, measles, and prolapses of the uterus, stomach, intestines, or bladder. They also believe it raises *chi*, the vital energy force.

The name *squaw root* comes from use by North American tribes to help facilitate labor. It was introduced to the medical world in 1844 by Dr. John King, who used it for rheumatism and nervous disorders. Black cohosh became a favorite herb with eclectic medical practitioners. It was widely used for scarlet fever, whooping cough, and smallpox. Herbalists have found that it improves blood circulation, lowers blood pressure and body temperature by dilating blood vessels, and depresses the central nervous system. One of the few remaining uses recognized by doctors today is relief of ringing ears. It has been found particularly useful for people suffering acute stages of rheumatoid arthritis. It relieves sinusitis and asthma, and it lowers cholesterol levels and blood pressure.

## TONIC USAGE
Black cohosh is a tall, leafy perennial native to North America. It grows abundantly in woods and on hillsides. It has a strong aroma and is a beautiful, graceful plant. However, there is a danger of overdose, which produces symptoms of vomiting, prostration, and reduced pulse. Pregnant women or those with heart problems should avoid this herb. For the tonic, use the rhizomes or roots, preferably from 2-year-old roots. The healing oil, however, is so resinous that it is more soluble in an alcohol-based tincture.

To make the tincture, dry and powder the root. Add ¼ cup of the powdered root to 1 pint of vodka. Close the jar tightly and shake every day, setting the jar in a sunny window for 2 weeks. Strain through a coffee filter or cheesecloth several times. Take 1 teaspoon of this tincture in 1 cup of hot water, sweetened with honey if preferred. Drink up to 3 cups per day.

## AVAILABILITY
Black cohosh can be purchased at some herb or health food shops. It is easy to grow if you have some wild open spaces.

# BORAGE

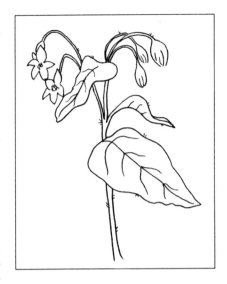

*Borago officinalis*
Also called burrage and common bugloss

## REPORTED BENEFITS

This herb once had the reputation for invoking courage. It produces feelings of elation and well-being. Borage has always been a favorite among soldiers, and ancient Celtic warriors prepared for battle by drinking wine flavored with it. Several noted herbalists and scholars have pointed out these qualities. The early Roman scholar Pliny thought the herb to be antidepressant. Dioscorides, the ancient Greek physician, wrote in his *De Materia Medica* that borage should be taken to cheer the heart and lift depressed spirits. The Welsh called it the herb of gladness. And Sir Francis Bacon wrote, "The leaf of burrage hath an excellent spirit to repress the fuliginous vapour of dusky melancholies." The Lebanese believed it to be an aphrodisiac. In the 17th century it was used for hypochondriacs. And the candied flowers were often given to cheer those recovering from long illnesses and to those prone to swooning.

Many early herbalists agree that it is helpful in relieving depression and it was once thought to relieve fevers. It has also been considered slightly diuretic, good for kidney and bladder inflammations, an astringent, and helpful in bronchitis, although slightly constipating. In Latin America, a tea made from borage was taken for rheumatism and other respiratory infections, as well as to restore vitality and calm.

## TONIC USAGE

Borage is an annual, with rough hairy leaves and pretty blue flowers shaped like stars. It is native to the Mediterranean region and self-seeds, growing from 1 to 3 feet. It blooms all summer and requires full sun. The taproot does not transplant well; so, it is best to seed it where you want it. Use the leaves and flowers, which have a faint cucumber taste. Some insist it is cooling, while others consider it spicy. The English novelist Charles Dickens was fond of borage punch and gave the recipe to American friends while visiting them. The flowers also taste great in salads.

When making a tea it is best to use borage dried since fresh borage is high in alkaloid content (similar to comfrey). Use 1 teaspoon in 1 cup of boiling water. Cover, steep 10 to 15 minutes, and strain. Also note that some people can have an allergic reaction, usually a rash, after handling the prickly leaves. You may want to wear gloves when harvesting it.

## AVAILABILITY
Borage seeds are readily available.

## CATNIP

*Nepeta cataria*
Also catmint and field balm

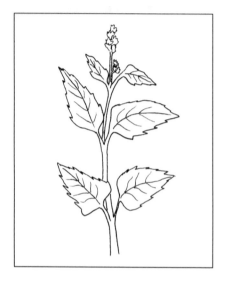

## REPORTED BENEFITS
Cats find catnip irresistible, and humans find it a mild relaxant, too, since it has a similar chemical structure to the well-known sedative valerian, although it's milder. One medicinal plant expert believes that the herb contains a hallucinogenic substance that also affects humans in some way. In fact, a 1960s article in the *Journal of the American Medical Association* caused quite a stir, since physicians claimed catnip did indeed have mild psychoactive properties. It was once used by hippies as a mild hallucinogen when smoked, but for health benefits one would use a tonic tea instead. Catnip is not a dangerous herb. In *The Honest Herbal* (1993), Varro Tyler, Ph.D., found evidence that the sedative qualities posed no harmful side effects. It was listed in the *U.S. Pharmacopeia* from 1842 to 1882.

Other medicinal uses for catnip include settling upset stomachs, soothing bronchitis, reducing flatulence and acidity, calming hysteria and nervousness, and relieving headaches. It contains tannins and a volatile oil with nepetalactone, a mild sedative that's good for helping you get a good night's sleep. Safe enough even for children to take, it increases body heat, stimulates perspiration, reduces fever, relieves hives, reduces hyperactivity, and even seems to quiet nightmares. It acts as a mild stimulant for digestion and appetite and relieves stress. In England, catnip was once a popular substitute for Chinese tea and was brought to America by the Colonists for this purpose. In France it was once considered a culinary seasoning, but now it is mainly cultivated in Europe and the Americas for manufacturing cat toys.

## TONIC USAGE

Catnip is a hardy spreading perennial that has a mintlike, bitter odor. This herb of the mint family self-seeds freely. Originally native to Europe, catnip is now found wild in the United States and Canada. It prefers sun or partial shade. The soft, heart-shaped leaves are downy gray. Pregnant women are advised not to drink large quantities of this tea. The taste is aromatic and minty. Use the leaves for your tonic tea; dry them on newspaper several days in a cool, dark place. To make the tea, add 2 teaspoons of dried or 1 tablespoon of fresh leaves to 1 cup of boiling water. Cover, steep 10 to 15 minutes, and strain. Drink up to 3 cups per day.

## AVAILABILITY

Catnip is readily available and easy to grow.

# CHAMOMILE

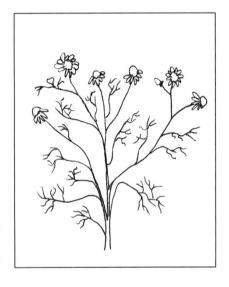

*Chamaemelum nobile* or *Anthemis nobilis*
Also called Roman chamomile

## REPORTED BENEFITS

The name *chamomile* means "ground apple," since when bruised or walked on, the herb has a pleasant applelike aroma. Chamomile was a favorite herb of the ancients. Egyptians believed it prevented aging, perhaps because of its ability to ease stress. Dioscorides and Pliny, great ancient herbalists, both advised use of chamomile for headaches; for kidney, liver, and bladder disorders; and for calming nerves and easing menstrual cramps and mild pains. It was also used as an anti-infective for minor ailments. It acts as a moderate sedative which soothes indigestion and stomach problems; it is also good for restless children. Some have asserted that the volatile oil content is so low it cannot be effective, but many herbalists disagree. Herbalist Rae Jean Elliott considers it is quite effective: "I truly believe that chamomile tops the list of renewing herbs. This herb can be used by almost anyone, from the youngest child to the oldest adult . . . It also helps to relieve anxiety, stress, and tension. In the business that I work in I am at times around chemicals. My eyelids can become red and sore, and get badly irritated on these days. However, when

I place chamomile tea bags on my eyes and lie down for 15 minutes, this is all it takes for me to find relief."

Chamomile has been recommended for hundreds of years to ease nerves and muscle pain. In one clinical study it was noted that 10 out of 12 patients who drank the tea instead of using regular pain medications were able to fall into a deep sleep within 10 minutes, even while undergoing a painful procedure. A pharmaceutical company in West Germany found that it reduces gastric acid and helps prevent ulcers, as well as decreases histamine production. Historically, poultices have been placed on cancers, and chamomile has been shown to stimulate the immune system and inhibit tumors. Some believe chamomile is high on the list for producing allergic reactions in those sensitive to ragweed. However, one study found that the likelihood of acute allergic reaction is very low, only 2 out of 25 people with allergies showing a reaction to chamomile. It is advised that you test your sensitivity if you are allergy-prone.

## TONIC USAGE

Chamomile is perennial and hardy. The leaves are light, bright green. It blooms with a yellow, daisylike flower June through July and grows 3 to 12 inches. It is a creeping, ground-cover herb that likes sun or takes partial shade. Use the flowers, which taste lightly of apple. Harvest the flowers and sprigs when the petals begin to turn back on the disk. Use fresh or dried, but dry the flowers and sprigs in a dark area spread out on newspapers until crumbly. Store the herb in a tightly covered jar. Use 2 teaspoons of dried or 1 tablespoon of fresh herb in 1 cup of boiling water. Cover and steep 20 minutes. Strain. If you use commercial tea bags, use 2 tea bags per cup. Drink up to 2 cups per day, but do not use chamomile over a long period. Drink it 2 weeks, rest 2 weeks, then begin again. Chamomile has been used as a lawn covering since Elizabethan times.

## AVAILABILITY

Chamomile is widely available, prepackaged in tea bags at gourmet and grocery stores. Commercially it is grown in Central Europe. The whole herb is used in beer manufacture.

# CLOVER

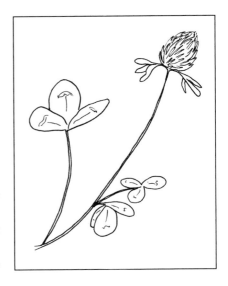

*Trifolium pratense*
Also called red clover and cowgrass

## REPORTED BENEFITS

In most places, this herb grows as a weed. But clover has a high protein content and is a favorite food for livestock and poultry. Humans have also long used it as a food source in a different way. Native North American tribes ate clover raw and cooked, but primarily the flowers were used fresh or dried in a tea for fevers, kidney ailments, and as a gynecological aid. The Iroquois used it for strenthening the blood. The high-protein leaves are a staple in China. In Europe and North America, it has been traditionally used as a blood purifier and has been considered one of the classic spring tonics.

Clover was originally included in the famous cancer remedy Hoxsey's Cure. Some interesting anticancer chemicals have been discovered in it, including antioxidants and other compounds. Researchers at Purdue University in Indiana found the results of their study on the herb's cancer-prevention activity significant enough to warrant further investigation. Several other laboratories have detected that clover contains compounds with estrogenic activity which may be helpful with breast cancer.

The herb is alterative, nutritive, and antispasmodic. It also acts as an expectorant and a mild sedative, often used with yellow dock or dandelion root. It stimulates the liver and gall bladder. Herbalists recommend it for detoxification, rebuilding, stimulation, and cleansing, and for creating a gradual sense of overall strengthening and nourishment. It has been used for gout, arthritis, skin disorders, and even AIDS. Antiasthma cigarettes which open the bronchial tubes were used until the 1970s and 1980s, when clover was replaced by newer, synthetic drugs. After clover cigarettes were replaced, asthma deaths increased, and it was discovered that the severity and frequency of asthma also increased in the long term, which in turn created a dependency on the manufactured drug. People with constipation or sluggish appetite were often advised to drink clover tea.

## TONIC USAGE

This short-lived perennial blooms July through August and prefers full sun, reaching up to 2 feet tall. It has compact flower heads, with three leaves on each stem. Use the flowers, which are full of nutrients, including vitamin C, most B vitamins, and minerals like magnesium, zinc, copper, and selenium. Use the blossoms fresh or dried; use the air-drying method rather than the oven. The taste of this tonic tea is delicate and sweet. Use 2 teaspoons of dried, chopped flowers or 1 tablespoon of fresh flowers per cup of boiling water. Steep 10 to 15 minutes. This tea is good with rose hips or mint.

## AVAILABILITY

Clover seeds can be found through farm seed-supply stores. It grows wild and is easy to identify.

# DILL

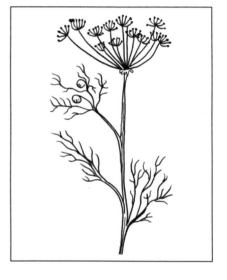

*Anethum graveolens*
Also called dillweed and dilly

## REPORTED BENEFITS

The name for dill in Old Norse, *dilla,* means "to lull," and that is exactly what dill was used for: inducing sleep. The seed decoction reduces insomnia and stomach pains, and quiets appetite. Herbalists use both leaves and seeds for flatulence and increasing mother's milk. It has also been used for breast congestion resulting from nursing. Dill oil kills bacteria and is frequently used in India's ayurvedic and unani medicines for a variety of ills. Ethiopians chew dill leaves along with fennel to treat headaches and even gonorrhea.

Dill has many historical and even biblical references, and it is still often included in children's medicines. Little dilly pillows were often used in European cradles to lull babies to sleep and to calm them with the scent. In the Middle Ages, it was believed that dill wine enhanced passion. American Colonists called it meeting-house seed, since they nibbled on dill seeds to prevent stomachs from rumbling in hunger during long hours in church. Nicholas Culpeper in *The Complete Herbal* (1649) listed dill as a "tonic that strengthens the braine." In the 19th century it became famous as a diet herb when a physician, Félix Pouchet, recommended that it be drunk as a thick broth each day. This excellent, safe tonic has been used to flavor foods, and it has slight stimulant actions.

## TONIC USAGE

The pungent smell will tell you that dill is growing nearby. It is a beautiful plant with feathery leaves; it looks like a smaller version of fennel. Dill, an annual growing 3 to 4 feet in the sun, has been naturalized in North America. Flowers appear July through September. To gather the seed wait until late summer or early fall, but leaves can be gathered in early summer. You can use dill fresh or dried, and the taste is tangy, sharp, and refreshing. The leaf is milder than the seed. To make a tonic tea from seed use 2 teaspoons of seed, added to 1 cup of boiling water. Steep 10 to 15 minutes and strain. If you prefer the leaves, add 1 teaspoon of dried leaves or 3 teaspoons fresh leaves to 1 cup of boiling water. Steep 5 to 10 minutes; drink 1 to 3 cups per day.

## AVAILABILITY

Dill is readily available fresh or dried at grocery stores and spice shops. It is easy to grow.

# HOP

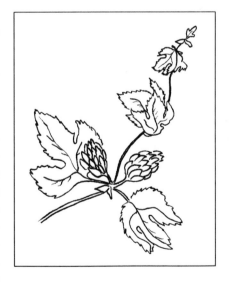

*Humulus lupulus*
Also called European hop, common hop, and bine

## REPORTED BENEFITS

Hops (the ripe dried pistillate catkins of the hop herb) revolutionized beer-brewing, enabling the brew to keep longer. It also causes the drowsiness often observed in beer drinkers. Traditionally, English doctors have used it to combat insomnia. In homeopathic medicine, hop has been used as a sedative and depurative, or purifier. Both American Abraham Lincoln and Englishman King George III are reported to have used sleep pillows made with hop. Many animals have been known to seek this herb out, including bees.

Experiments done with frogs, birds, and mice show that hop does depress the central nervous system. It has always been regarded as a bitter tonic. Herbalists report that hop increases vital energy and the vigor of organs, although one can overdose on it. Symptoms include heavy, tired limbs, quickened pulse, raised body heat, and even vomiting. The female flower tea contains lupulin, a mild narcotic; so, because of both its narcotic qualities and the possibility of overdosing, prolonged use of hop tonic is not advised.

Hop has often been used in combination with other herbs as a mild sedative, weak diuretic, and weak antibiotic. It has been helpful with ulcers, irritable bowel syndrome, and Crohn's disease, and used as an aid for nervous indigestion. At one time hop was used to treat prostate disorders. Hop has been found to relax nerves and smooth muscles (especially in the digestive tract), and it reacts quite quickly, within 20 to 40 minutes, after ingestion. A 1980 study found that hop contains a muscle relaxant in addition to lupulin. Also contained within hop are estrogenlike compounds. These compounds were discovered when pickers gathering female hop cones noticed changes in their menstrual cycles after absorbing the essential oils through their hands. Aphrodisiac effects were observed in male pickers, although its narcotic properties have, paradoxically, made it useful in controlling sexual desire. Regular doses can help regulate the menstrual cycle. It also contains gamma-linoleic acid, which also occurs in evening primrose; this makes it useful for premenstrual syndrome, muscle cramps, headaches, and sore breasts. It has been used for restlessness, stress, circulation, and shock. Regular doses may even decrease the desire for alcohol.

## TONIC USAGE

Hop grows wild and has been cultivated in northern Europe, the United States, Canada, and Chile. It is a tall, spindly, clinging vine that reaches up to 30 feet. It has bright green leaves, but the flowers and cones are used. The flowers appear midsummer, sometimes growing up to 11 inches long. Use fresh flowers or cones for your tonic, since a study demonstrated that 85 percent of the original chemical vitality was lost over a 9-month storage period. For winter use, make a tincture. Place a handful of the flower or cones into vodka; steep 1 week in a sunny window. Strain and add more plant material, repeating these steps until the liquid is a strong yellow color. Use ½ teaspoon of this liquid per cup of hot water. In using fresh flowers and cones, take 1 tablespoon and add it to ½ pint of water, bring the tea to a boil, then simmer 2 to 3 minutes. Steep covered for 15 minutes and then strain. The tea tastes slightly peppery, yet mild, and it has a light yellow color. Drink 1 to 2 cups over a 3- to 4-day period.

## AVAILABILITY
Hop can be purchased where dried herbs are sold. It is easy to grow if you have trellis space.

# LAVENDER

*Lavandula angustifolia*

## REPORTED BENEFITS
Famous for its fresh, clean scent, lavender is believed to help cure insomnia, nervousness, heart palpitations, halitosis, gas, fainting, and dizziness. Victorian women prone to fainting often sniffed hankies scented with this herb to revive themselves. During the Middle Ages, it was considered an aphrodisiac, but people also sprinkled lavender water over the head to keep themselves chaste. British herbalist

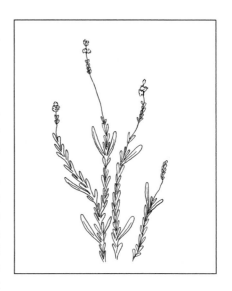

Maude Grieve mentions it for digestion. Herbalists claim its powers are as a carminative, antispasmodic, and stimulant. It is also a wonderful burn-healer, and in some parts of Europe, lavender has been used to quiet coughs and rumbling digestive systems. A compound tincture of this herb, also known as palsy drops, and listed in the *British Pharmacopoeia* until 1940, was used for muscle spasms, nervousness, and headaches. A particular species, *Lavandula stoechas*, has been used in early stages of paralysis and for epilepsy, with some success.

Little scientific work has been done on the plant, but the few studies have indicated that it is valuable as a medicinal. In China, lavender is used in a cure-all medicinal oil called white flower oil. Tests show it is potent as an antibacterial good for flu, viruses, and strep. It is also strongly antifungal and can be used as a douche for yeast infections or applied to itchy insect bites. The whole plant is relaxing and acts as a sedative and tonic. Lavender is still used in folk medicines internally as a mild sedative, a cough suppressant, and for gastric disturbances. The fragrance has been said to mentally relax and also to raise the spirits.

## TONIC USAGE
Lavender is a wonderfully scented flower, a perennial growing 1½ to 3 feet, with woody upright stems and narrow leaves with blue blooms. It flowers

from July through September and is difficult to start from seed. The tea is cooling and sweetly aromatic and flowery. Pick the blossom buds before they open, and strip them from the stems. You can also use the leaves of the plant. To dry, spread out on newspapers in a darkened room until crumbly. To make a tonic tea, use 1 teaspoon of dried leaves or 3 teaspoons of fresh leaves to 1 cup of boiling water, cover, and steep 5 to 10 minutes. Strain. This is a very safe tea, but do use it in moderation, up to 3 cups per day.

## AVAILABILITY
Lavender is readily available dried at any shops that sell dried herbs. The plant is somewhat tricky to grow.

# LEMON BALM

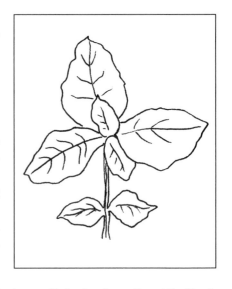

*Melissa officinalis*
Also called balm mint, bee balm, and honey balm

## REPORTED BENEFITS
Common to the Mediterranean region and the Near East, this wonderful herb has naturalized itself in the United States and Canada, where it grows wild in fields and gardens and along roadsides. American Colonists used it to lift their spirits; Thomas Jefferson grew it at Monticello. Lemon balm was regarded mainly as a bee plant until the Arabs took an interest in its medicinal values. Specifically, it has been used for anxiety, depression, and as a sedative and tonic to reduce colic, cramps, bronchial congestion, migraine headaches, dizziness, nausea, stomachaches, restlessness, and some forms of asthma. The tea is a wonder, like no other for dispelling melancholy and sadness. It is both calming yet stimulating. Lemon balm acts as a tranquilizer and was used as a mild form of Valium in past centuries. It relaxes heart spasms, lowers blood pressure, and is helpful when appetite is lacking. It is gentle enough for children yet still very potent. Herbalists have used it for colds, fevers, and flus to bring on sweats, and as an antiviral agent good against mumps, cold sores, and other viruses.

The Muslim herbalist Avicenna (980–1037) recommended it "to make the heart merry." Paracelsus claimed that it could completely revitalize the

114

body. The 14th century French King Charles V drank it every day to maintain his health. Lemon balm was the chief ingredient in the famous Carmelite water, made by 17th century Carmelite nuns to treat nervous headaches. The true Carmelite water is still sold in Germany as *Klosterfrau Melissengeist*. Mental disorders have been calmed by this herb, especially restlessness, excitability, or headaches. Studies indicate that it slightly inhibits thyroid-stimulating hormone and restricts Grave's disease, a hyperthyroid condition. It also has antihistamine action that's useful for eczema and insect bites. Since the essential oil is quite expensive, it is often replaced with citronella oil. If you buy the oil, make sure you're getting pure lemon balm.

## TONIC USAGE
Much of the value of this essential oil is lost in drying; so, for winter use, it's best to make a tincture. This perennial herb has an intense lemony smell and grows 1½ to 4 feet tall in sun or partial shade. Lemon balm is very easy to grow, self-seeding, and spreading. If you don't have the space or inclination, you can purchase the essential oil. If you do choose to grow it yourself, you can make a leaf tea which is lemony and quite refreshing.

Gather the leaves in the early morning after the dew has dried. Use 1 tablespoon of the leaves added to 1 cup of boiling water. Steep 10 minutes. To use the essential oil, add 2 to 4 drops to a cup of hot water, mix, and drink. To make your own tincture, put a handful of fresh leaves in a quart jar. Add enough vodka to cover the leaves, and set the jar in a sunny window 1 to 2 weeks. Remove the plant material and add fresh leaves, repeating the procedure until the liquid smells strongly of lemon. Add 1 teaspoon of this to a cup of boiling water. Drink 2 to 3 cups per day.

## AVAILABILITY
Lemon balm essential oil is expensive but lasts a long time. The plant is also easy to grow yourself.

# SKULLCAP

*Scutellaria laterifolia*
Also called mad-dog weed and Virginia skullcap

## REPORTED BENEFITS
Skullcap was once thought to cure rabies, but it also found its way into many 19th century patent medicines as a nerve tonic and remedy for epilepsy. The leaves are used mostly for their action on the nervous system,

specifically anxiety, depression, insomnia, nervous headaches, twitches, muscle cramps, and convulsions. The herb is good for rheumatism, pain, and stress; it also improves circulation, strengthens the heart muscle, and aids sleep. Eclectic 19th century doctors found it helpful for nervousness due to emotional stress or physical exhaustion and used it as a bitter to stimulate digestion.

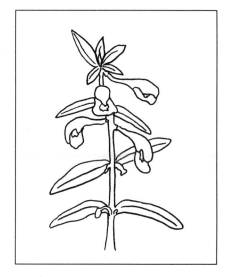

Few scientific studies have been done on this particular species. Russian research supports the usefulness of skullcap as a sedative and stabilizer of stress-related heart disease, since they've shown that it lowers blood pressure and cholesterol. Many native North American tribes knew its soothing qualities and used it for heart problems and to regularize menstruation. Herbalist Michael Tierra has found it helpful in treating drug and alcohol withdrawal symptoms. Clinical studies with skullcap (*Scutellaria baicalensis*) in China found it improved symptoms in over 70 percent of those with chronic hepatitis. It increased the appetite, improved liver function, and reduced swelling and allergic reactions.

## TONIC USAGE
Since large doses can cause mental confusion and dizziness, use care in dosage. This herb is native to the United States, Newfoundland, and British Columbia. This perennial can take partial shade and it spreads slowly. For a tonic tea, use the leaves and stems, which contain fat, iron, glycoside, and vitamin E. Dry the plant material on newspapers in a dark place. The tea tastes bitter; so, you may want to add honey or other herbs to your brew. Take 1 ounce of the dried herb and pour boiling water (1¼ pints) over it. Cover and steep 20 minutes. Strain. Drink ½ teacup at bedtime and drink no more than a full cup in a day.

## AVAILABILITY
Dried skullcap is available at health food or herb stores.

# VALERIAN

*Valeriana officinalis*

## REPORTED BENEFITS

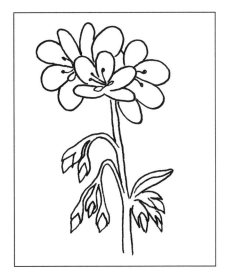

The Roman name of the herb *valere* was derived from the word *valor*, meaning "courage," since courage was needed to drink the stinky brew! Galen and Dioscorides called the herb *phu*, describing its odor. If it were not for valerian's many powerful medicinal uses, the smell would surely keep us away. It has been used as a general tranquilizer and as an insomnia and headache remedy. This wonderful renewing herb has been widely studied and shown to sedate the central nervous system. Herbalist Harriett Prosperi adds: "Valerian has been very useful for the people who have asked me for help in sleeping and relaxing."

Indeed, many have been impressed. Herbalists note that valerian decreases muscle spasms, nervous digestion, irritable bowel syndrome, and stomach and menstrual cramps. The herb contains substances of opposing effects that apparently allow it to regulate many conditions. In one study, it sedated agitated patients but stimulated those fatigued. In another study, it improved the quality of the subjects' sleep, and reduced the time it took for them to fall asleep. It was particularly effective for the elderly and habitually poor sleepers. The herb did not interfere with dream recall or patients' ability to awaken the next morning, in contrast with many pharmaceutical sleep aids, which have side effects. It can also be taken with alcohol without the appearance of depression often associated with alcohol consumption along with tranquilizers. It has been considered a psychological drug which affects the central nervous system.

In Germany, hyperactive children have been treated with this herb since the 1970s. Valerian has proven very helpful in lessening aggressive behavior, restlessness, fear, and anxiousness, and it has helped the learning disabled with muscle coordination. Animal studies have indicated that it may lower blood pressure and strengthen optic nerves. Valerian and its derivatives were marketed in West Germany in over a hundred proprietary drugs. However after centuries of use in the United States, including inclusion in the *U.S. Pharmacopoeia* from 1820 to 1942 and in the *U.S. National Formulary* from 1942 until 1950 as a tranquilizer, valerian-based drugs are not now available. It has been used since ancient times and by English herbalists John Gerard and Nicholas Culpeper in the 16th and 17th centuries.

## TONIC USAGE

In the medicinal tea, the roots or rhizomes are used. In 1907 research found fresh valerian more active than the dried root, but that is perhaps true of any herb. Since it is powerful, do not use this herb during pregnancy. Avoid prolonged or large dosages since this will cause headaches, muscle spasms, and heart palpitations.

This leafy herb has a tall flowering stalk and grows up to 5 feet. The roots smell like dirty socks. It blooms in early to midsummer. The native habitat is Europe and western Asia, but the herb now grows in Canada and the northern United States. This perennial can be found in low meadows and wet woods and requires partial shade. Harvest only second-year roots. You can deflower young plants to hasten root development. Dig the roots in fall or spring before shoots sprout. Wash, slice thinly, then dry quickly in a low oven (120° F) until brittle. The roots will keep the odor and flavor a long time.

It will be hard to drink the tea unless you mix it with other sweet herbs. To prepare it, pour 1 pint of boiling water over 1 teaspoon of powdered root. Cover, steep 15 minutes, then strain. If you wish, you can make a tincture of the root. Drink 1 cup at bedtime per day and be prepared to sleep.

## AVAILABILITY

Seed can be obtained from specialty herb seed carriers. You can also purchase the dried root.

# Regenerative or Alterative Tonic Herbs

*Alterative herbs,* herbs which alter the disease process and aid in renewal, are useful for people who have weakened immune systems, endured a long illness, or continue to suffer severe disease. These herbs are capable of regenerating the body's weakened immune system.

When in the early 1920s Harry Hoxsey claimed he had a cure for cancer in a remedy consisting merely of herbs found in the wild, simple weeds with healing properties, the American medical community was not happy about it. They fought to suppress the wondrous elixir and called Hoxsey's Cure a hoax. Hoxsey struggled to prove his claims and eventually opened over 17 cancer clinics across the United States by the 1950s. And thousands of cancer patients claimed to have been cured by Hoxsey's Cure. The U.S. Food & Drug Administration eventually closed down his clinics and succeeded in discrediting folk healing or "weed healing," as they called it.

This dealt a blow to herbal healing in the United States that herbalists and patients have just begun to recover from. Herbs represent an alternative choice. They offer hope for a stronger, healthier, renewed body. All the herbs discussed in these chapters—blood purifiers, immune-system strengtheners, vitamin-packed antioxidants, and milder rejuvenators—help renew and strengthen the body. However, herbs called alterative have a special job, too. Alterative herbs are overall strengtheners and detoxifiers that are similar to other tonic herbs, but they specifically direct the body toward recovery from illness. This means that the body gains support in its most weakened state.

Mildred Nelson, director of the Bio-Medical Center in Mexico (using the same formula and healing method as in Hoxsey's original clinics), claims an 80 percent cancer cure rate. Orthodox medical therapies do not approach this rate with chemotherapy, radiation, and surgery.

Medicinal herbs have in many documented cases succeeded when conventional treatments failed. Some patients have used herbs during or before beginning traditional medical treatments. According to legend, long ago a wise herbal teacher in India asked his students to gather and bring him all the plants they could find that had no medicinal use. The students searched and brought back various herbs, but one student returned with nothing. He told the wise teacher he could not find a single plant that could not be used in healing. The teacher praised him and said he alone was prepared to be a physician.

Here are ten alterative herbs to add to your herbal repertoire.

# BAYBERRY

*Myrica cerifera*
Also called wax myrtle and candle-
berry

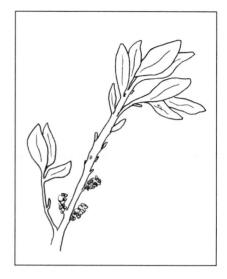

## REPORTED BENEFITS
Bayberry, a simple-looking perennial
shrub, has been used in folk medicine
as a tonic. The leaves, bark, and roots
have stimulant and astringent properties. The tea was used for sore throats,
spongy gums, and jaundice. The
leaves have also been used in the
same culinary way as the tropical bay
leaves you buy at the store. It was also
used as a source for wax in Colonial America. The berries are covered with
wax which was melted and collected for use in candlemaking and soap-
making. Old-time herbalists have used this herb as a snuffing powder to
cure congestion and nasal polyps.

Today, it is used as an alterative with slight narcotic properties. Studies
have shown it to be effective in ulcerated conditions of the throat and gums.
It improves circulation, tones the gastrointestinal tissues, and clears sinus
congestion. It helps diarrhea and dyspepsia and acts as a stimulant for
sluggish liver function. It contains myricitrin, which kills pathogenic bacteria and promotes the flow of bile.

## TONIC USAGE
This tonic should be used over short periods of time. The shrubs are
attractive, with aromatic berries. Bayberry grows widely across the United
States as a wild plant, but can be easily cultivated and requires little care as
long as it is planted in the sun. It even survives in poor sandy soils. The plant
flowers in early spring and berries appear in midsummer.

It is a bitter tonic similar to goldenseal and Oregon grape. In the fall dig
the root and strip the bark. Then chop, dry, and powder it, and store it in
a tightly closed jar. In a 1970 study, rats were injected with bark extract for
78 weeks, and after that time the animals were found to have developed
cancerous tumors; so, do not use it on a long-term basis. Often in nature,
plants have countereffects. Many herbs reported to cure cancer have also
been found to cause it when used in excess. Nature apparently demands
balance in everything.

The leaves are the weakest part of the plant and should be used for less
severe conditions. Use 2 teaspoons of crushed fresh leaves (or 1 teaspoon of
120

dried), and add this to 1 cup of boiling water. Steep 10 to 15 minutes, strain, and drink up to 3 cups per day. To use the powdered root bark, add 1 tablespoon per cup of water. Bring to a boil, then reduce heat, and simmer for 10 minutes. Do not strain, but stir well before drinking. Drink up to 2 cups per day. You may wish to mix with other, sweeter herbs or add honey. In some people, it may initially cause nausea and slight pain which will pass, and the stimulant actions will then take effect.

## AVAILABILITY
Dried root bark can be purchased. The bayberry plant is easy to grow.

# GARLIC

*Allium sativum*

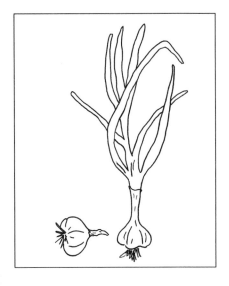

## REPORTED BENEFITS
Garlic, prized as a favorite medicinal plant, was believed by the ancients to strengthen the body and prevent many diseases. It was listed in ancient Egyptian scrolls as a medicinal herbal along with about 800 other herbs. According to the Greek historian Herodotus, garlic was eaten for endurance by slaves who constructed the Cheops pyramid. It was also found in King Tut's tomb. Historically, it has been used to treat leprosy, and diseases which cause pus to form on any part of the body have been reportedly cured when garlic was applied to the soles of the feet.

Garlic was an important ingredient in the famous tonic Four Thieves' Vinegar, used by four 14th century thieves to protect themselves from the plague as they robbed houses. Garlic is a universal antiseptic. During outbreaks of infectious fever in London, French priests who used garlic in all their dishes did not become sick, while the English clergy who shunned garlic often fell ill. The Indian herbalist Charaka from the 1st century A.D. claimed garlic would one day be worth its weight in gold.

Louis Pasteur observed its antibacterial effects in 1858, and by the second half of the 20th century, more than 1,000 scientific papers were published on garlic's use in fighting infection and lowering blood cholesterol.

Allicin, the active chemical in garlic, is indeed powerful. In a 1950 study, Dr. J. Klosa found that 15 to 25 drops of garlic oil, given every 4 hours, had the ability to kill dangerous organisms, without attacking more helpful vital organisms as penicillin does. He found it effective with flu. In 71 cases of subjects with clogged and runny noses, 100 percent found their symptoms gone within 13 to 20 minutes.

Herbalists report that it cures tuberculosis, asthma, skin diseases, and stomach ulcers and restores health to a weakened body. It is specific for the respiratory system and may be used as a germicide, to disinfect, and as an expectorant and a nervine. Garlic discourages viruses and bacteria like staphylococcus or Escherichia coli.

In Chinese clinical studies, it cured 67 percent of a group with intestinal bacterial infections and 88 percent with amebic dysentery. Also, study subjects who ate garlic for 6 months had significantly lower blood cholesterol and fat levels. Researchers have noted success in treating fungal infections, whooping cough, lead poisoning, and some carcinomas. Garlic dramatically activates the immune system and many studies suggest that it inhibits tumors. Residents in one region of China who do not eat garlic have 1,000 times higher rates of stomach cancer than those of the garlic-eating regions. Even appendicitis was improved in a few studies.

Another study found that garlic detoxified harmful lead levels in the blood, and has suggested that garlic actually prevents accumulations of toxins. Many cultures have noted that it helps control mild diabetes. It thins the blood by inhibiting platelet aggregation, reducing blood clots and preventing heart attacks. Garlic is noted for its ability to reduce blood pressure without depleting the body of vital minerals as many conventional medicines do. It is also effective for inflammations, such as arthritis, and for circulation problems.

## TONIC USAGE

According to folk wisdom, garlic should be eaten every day, and there is no harm in doing so. This annual from the onion family can be easily grown in the garden and prefers full sun. It contains vitamins A, $B_1$, $B_2$, C, and various minerals. Use the bulb, which is also the part used for centuries for flavor in cooking. For tonic usage, the fresher, the better; so use oil from cloves rather than dried powder. Garlic has been used in decoctions in the form of syrups, juice, tinctures, or poultices, and today it is used in both veterinary and homeopathic medicine. Many find it disagreeable because of the "garlicky" smell it produces in the breath. Fennel seeds or parsley leaves will take away the odor; so, you may want to use these herbs with it.

To make a tonic, add 1 cup of sliced cloves to 1 pint of olive oil or vinegar. Soak them in a sunny window 1 week, shaking occasionally. Strain and refrigerate. Add ½ teaspoon of this mixture to a warm tonic tea, up to three doses per day. You can use the garlic daily as long as you wish.

## AVAILABILITY
Garlic is readily available at grocery stores and produce markets.

# GENTIAN

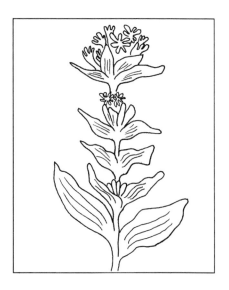

*Gentiana lutea*
Also called bitter root or yellow gentian

## REPORTED BENEFITS
This herb contains one of the most bitter substances ingested by humans. You can reduce its bitterness by using dried material, but it will still remain extremely bitter. Because of its bitterness, digestive juices flow within 5 minutes after the herb reaches the stomach. If taken 30 to 60 minutes before eating, gentian increases the appetite, stimulates digestive juices and pancreas activity, and increases the blood supply to the digestive tract, thereby decreasing intestinal inflammation. A German study found it extremely effective in curing indigestion and heartburn. It has been used to treat liver and spleen disorders. Since it promotes menstruation, do *not* use it when pregnant. Gentian is helpful for gout and arthritis.

King Gentius of Illyria (180 to 67 B.C.) introduced gentian as a medicinal when it cured his army of a mysterious fever. Gentian was an ingredient in eternal youth elixirs. Today, it is the chief flavoring in vermouth, Stoughton, and Angostura Bitters, both originally digestive tonics. This alterative herb stores vast quantities of oxygen in its roots, which causes it to be bitter, and seems to hold miraculous healing properties, especially when the body has excessive toxic wastes or is very ill. Chronic disease and debility can be greatly helped, and herbalists rank it as one of the best herbs for strengthening or building the human body. It mixes well with other herbs and is a modifier. If combined with a diuretic herb, it can modify and prevent the system from losing too much fluid or becoming weakened.

## TONIC USAGE
This 3-foot perennial has yellow flowers and a thick taproot. It flowers in early summer and likes cool, moist, shady locations. It hails from mountainous regions in France and Switzerland, but has been commercially

cultivated in eastern Europe and North America. It is difficult to establish, but once you do, the plants can live up to 50 years. Sow fresh seed in autumn. Established plants can be divided.

Herbalists use the root; the tonic should be taken 1 hour before eating. Harvest the root in the fall, slice and dry it slowly, then powder it. If you purchase gentian, the color should be dark reddish brown. It has a strong odor, with a taste that is sharp or sweet, with a bitter bite. Use 1½ to 2 ounces of powder in 1 pint of boiling water. Cover and steep 20 minutes and then strain. You can add 1 pint of honey to make a syrup. Add 2 teaspoons per cup of warm water; stir well. Drink up to 3 cups per day.

## AVAILABILITY
Gentian is readily available at health food stores.

# GINSENG

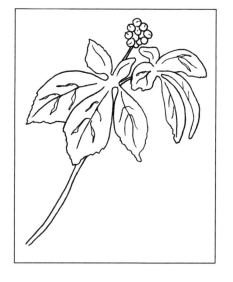

*Panax quinquefolius*
Also called American ginseng and man root

## REPORTED BENEFITS
Ginseng is popular as a whole-body tonic, and it is a legendary aphrodisiac. This herb boasts a 2,000-year history as an herb that prolongs life and as a cure for many human ills. The Chinese herbal *shen-nung pent-ts'ao-ching* from the 1st century A.D. includes it as a medicinal. And the Chinese have long attributed to the root the power of giving long life and wisdom. Wars were fought between the Chinese and Tartars over ginseng-growing territories. Ginseng and Virginia snakeroot made up the bulk of Virginia's medicinal exports in the early 1700s. The Shakers included it in many of their tonics.

Most researchers agree that ginseng protects the body against physical and mental stress. In one study, when subjects took ⅛ ounce of ginseng with alcohol, their blood alcohol level was as much as 51 percent lower than that of a control group consuming the same amount of alcohol. This suggests that ginseng helps the body functions return to normal more quickly, thereby increasing physical endurance. This can be quite useful for someone weakened by sickness. A 1957 study demonstrated increased endurance and concentration levels. Ginseng is often combined with other herbs, and herbalists use it readily in a great many different situations. It appears to help counteract aging effects and can be helpful for strengthening the body after surgery or severe stress. Western pharmacologists have even created a new term, *adaptogen*, to explain normalizing effects on the body which ginseng creates. For example, it has a dual role of sedating or stimulating the central nervous system, depending upon the body's needs.

## TONIC USAGE

The plant grows 1 to 2 feet tall from a single stem. It is a perennial with bright red berries that prefers cool, damp, shady spots like woodlands. The root is used medicinally, and its wrinkled shape resembles a human body. It takes 4 to 6 years for the roots to be fully mature. At one time, ginseng grew wild in the eastern United States and parts of Canada, but it is rapidly becoming endangered because of its popularity. Ginseng has now become a cultivated crop in North America that brings great profits. China continues to cultivate it. At one time, Russians were researching an herb with similar properties. The Chinese root is thought the most potent.

Collect the root only in autumn; rinse and chop it into pieces. Dry completely. Add 1 tablespoon of the chopped root to 1 pint of water. Bring to a boil and simmer 30 minutes. Strain. Drink ½ cup twice a day. This herb should not be taken in large doses.

## AVAILABILITY

It is available in health food stores. But make sure you purchase commercially grown ginseng to help keep it from disappearing from the wild.

Although it requires long-term growth, cultivating ginseng in your backyard can eventually pay off.

# HAWTHORN

*Crataegus laevigata*
Also called mayblossom, English hawthorn, and white thorn

## REPORTED BENEFITS

Ancient Greeks and Romans regarded this herb as the symbol of hope and happiness. And it does restore hope to heart patients. It acts directly on the heart muscle, helping a damaged heart work more efficiently. But the herb works slowly and serves as a mild tonic. This makes it a potentially important heart medication source since it dilates blood vessels, allowing blood to flow freely and lowering blood pressure. Studies show that hawthorn increases enzyme activity in the heart muscle to increase health and oxygen utilization. It even works well with digitalis, though a physician may need to halve the dosage. The herb works over a long period of time without the side effects of digitalis. It also has diuretic properties.

Scientific studies conclude that hawthorn is effective against hardening of the arteries. Studies have found that the flowers in full bloom and young leaves contain the most active ingredients and are antibiotic. The berries contain vitamin C. Early herbalists have also used it for kidney ailments, insomnia, and stress, and for relieving abdominal distension and diarrhea. Its special healing powers are believed to have come from its having been the crown of thorns Christ wore. It acts as an adaptogenic agent like garlic.

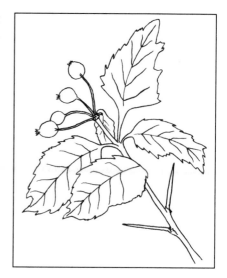

## TONIC USAGE

Hawthorn is a deciduous shrub or tree with thorny branches that grows up to 15 feet. It thrives along woodland edges in North America, Europe, and North Africa. It will grow in sun or partial shade. There have been berry decoctions and syrups made, but the flowers and young leaves are strongest. Use either or add them together. The flowers and leaves have a flat, astringent taste; the berries are tart or sweet.

To make a tonic tea, use 2 teaspoons of the chopped flowers and leaves for 1 cup of boiling water. Cover and steep 10 to 15 minutes. To use the berries, add 1 teaspoon dried or 2 teaspoons of crushed fresh fruit to 1 cup of water. Bring to a boil, reduce heat, simmer 15 minutes, then strain. You may drink up to 2 cups per day.

## AVAILABILITY

You can purchase the dried berries from places that sell dried herbs. For fresh flowers and leaves, you'll have to grow your own.

# PAU D'ARCO

*Tabebuia impetiginosa*
Also called lapacho and taheebo

## REPORTED BENEFITS

As a healing herb, pau d'arco has caused excitement. Researchers in the United States have even been exploring its use for cancer treatment, based on the findings of doctors in South America, who have used it to successfully treat leukemia and other cancers. It is an antibacterial agent and blood cleanser. Herbalists have found it useful for smoker's cough, warts, infections, diabetes, ulcers, arthritis, allergies, tumors, AIDS, leukemia, cancer, and liver disease. It has been recognized as an important herb for uses in autoimmune diseases, glandular disorders, and other serious health problems.

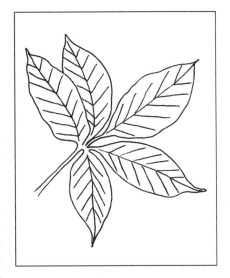

Though it is a strong alterative herb, it poses no side effects and can be easily mixed with other herbs to make tonic mixtures. Ancient Mayans used it to cure a variety of health problems and to build and strengthen the whole system.

## TONIC USAGE
A tender perennial, pau d'arco grows wild in the rain forests of South America, and as a rain forest plant, its survival is tenuous. Be sure to purchase only organically, commercially grown material.

Harvest the inner bark, chop, and dry. Use 4 to 6 tablespoons per quart of water and bring to a boil. Reduce heat, simmer for 20 minutes, then strain. Drink up to 3 cups per day and use for a maximum of 3 to 6 months at a time.

## AVAILABILITY
The dried bark is available in most herb and natural food stores.

# ROSEMARY

*Rosmarinus officinalis*

## REPORTED BENEFITS
In Latin *rosmarinus* means "dew of the sea"; later the herb was called rose of Mary in honor of the Virgin. The ancients believed it strengthened memory, restored youth, stimulated the heart, and induced sleep. In the 16th century, Europeans carried it to ward off the plague and other diseases. Rosemary is a traditional European treatment for people suffering poor circulation due to

illness or lack of exercise. Until recently, the scent was used to purify the air in French hospitals.

Studies show that rosemary increases circulation, reduces headaches, fights bacterial and fungal infections, and has the ability to strengthen fragile blood vessels. It also improves food absorption by stimulating digestion, as well as the liver, intestinal tract, and gallbladder. It inhibits stone formation in the bladder and kidneys. Researchers have found it good as a treatment for septic shock. In one laboratory study it was found to inhibit 87 percent of the cancer cells

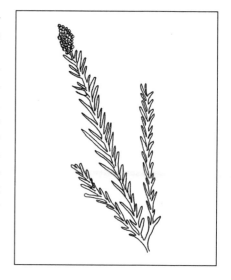

tested. Herbalists consider rosemary a tonic and find it helpful in depression and muscle spasms. The oil is included in the *U.S. Pharmacopeia,* and the whole herb remains popular in folk medicine. It promotes menstruation and is a strong stimulant. Avoid it if you are pregnant.

## TONIC
Rosemary is a graceful shrub, a tender perennial which blooms in early summer. Originating from the Mediterranean region, it takes full sun or partial shade. It grows wild and can be cultivated and used as a culinary herb. It tastes pinelike, but pleasant. To make a tonic tea, use the leaves and flowers' young tender tips. Add ½ teaspoon of fresh or 1 teaspoon of dried material per cup of boiling water. Cover and steep 10 to 15 minutes.

## AVAILABILITY
Rosemary is readily available fresh or dried.

# SAGE

*Salvia officinalis*
Also called common sage or garden sage

## REPORTED BENEFITS
Old herbals expressed the belief that sage was helpful to grieving patients, strengthening them mentally and physically. They also claimed it restored health to those with "palsy." It has been used for throat inflammations. An old English proverb states, "He that would live for aye, must eat sage in May."

The term *salvia* comes from a Latin word meaning "to save," which refers to its healing properties. Sage was a staple of old-time herbalists and many did indeed believe it prolonged life.

Today, we know that sage has stimulant properties, and acts as a tonic, a digestive, and an antiseptic. It also checks sweats. In one study, it reduced sweating by half within 2 hours of ingesting the herb. It lowers blood sugar production in diabetics when taken on an empty stomach. In a 1939 experiment sage showed some estrogenic properties, and this is why it was recommended in folk medicine for 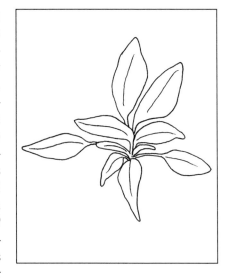 women who wanted to dry up milk when they had an infection or other breast problem. It has been used in many compound drugs, and in Germany an antiperspirant contains it. It is a strong antioxidant with antibacterial qualities. It fights cold germs and flu. Studies also show it is effective against staph infections.

## TONIC USAGE
This hardy perennial with gray-green leaves prefers full sun but can take partial shade. It grows 2 to 3 feet tall and flowers bloom midsummer, appearing on tall spikes. Sage is a cultivated herb used extensively in cooking as a flavoring. The leaves, which are highly aromatic, are used. Sage has a camphorlike, slightly bitter taste. To make a tonic tea, add 3 to 4 tablespoons of dried material or 4 to 5 tablespoons of fresh material to 1 quart of boiling water. Cover and steep 15 to 20 minutes. You can drink up to 3 cups per day.

## AVAILABILITY
Sage is readily available.

# SLIPPERY ELM

*Ulmus rubra*
Also called red elm and Indian elm

## REPORTED BENEFITS
The moist, slippery inner bark gives this tree its name. North American tribes used slippery elm as a tea to treat diarrhea or as a laxative, depending upon the need. This alterative herb suits many different health situations. It

is mucilaginous and safe, and is good against any mucous membrane inflammations or irritations.

It is used commercially to make nutritive convalescent drinks since it helps clear congestion. This mild diuretic is a wonderful strengthener that's also soothing. It has been helpful in asthma, bronchitis, lung ailments (checks coughing and heals bleeding lungs), and heart disease. It eases pain, spasms, distress, and exhaustion. It has been found useful in treating cystitis. Slippery elm can be tolerated by the stomach when nothing else can be.

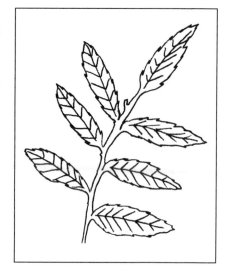

## TONIC USAGE
This small to medium tree has dark green leaves and ranges from North America to southern Canada. It grows wild in most woodlands and along streams. To make a healing tea, use the inner bark, collected in the spring. It smells slightly like fenugreek. If you buy the powdered bark, it should be gray or fawn colored. Collect the bark, dry and powder it. Mix 1 teaspoon with 1 tablespoon of cold water to a jellylike consistency. Add this to 1 pint of boiling water. You can drink up to 3 cups per day; sweeten with honey if you wish.

## AVAILABILITY
The powdered bark is available.


# ST.-JOHN'S-WORT

*Hypericum perforatum*

## REPORTED BENEFITS
In 1977 St.-John's-wort was placed on the "unsafe" herb list by the U.S. Food & Drug Administration because animals ingesting it developed a phototoxic reaction when exposed to the sun. No cases of human poisoning exist, however, and the herb has been attributed with many healing qualities as long as the dosage is kept low. Both pills and the extract are used today in homeopathy. Studies show it is a potent antiviral and antibacterial

agent. It contains over 50 constituents, some of which have been found helpful in treating herpes simplex, flu, and possibly even AIDS and cancer, according to researchers. One clinical study demonstrated that women experienced significant relief from anxiety symptoms after 4 to 6 weeks of taking the extract.

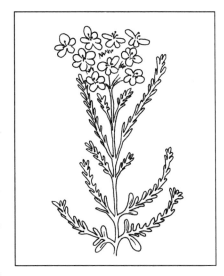

Herbalists claim that St.-John's-wort is helpful for depression and disturbed sleep patterns. It repairs nerve damage, reduces pain and inflammation, and relieves menstrual cramps, arthritis, circulation problems, gout, and incontinence. Its pain-relieving properties and ability to help prevent hemorrhaging make it helpful in recovery after surgery. The tea strengthens the immune system and is a strong alterative herb, although it can cause sun sensitivity. Care should be taken in using it. Monitor dosage and avoid sunlight. Also do not use the herb if you have sensitive skin.

## TONIC USAGE
This many-branched perennial rises from ground runners and grows 2 to 3 feet tall. It has star-shaped yellow flowers which bloom midsummer. It likes full sun or semishade. Propagate it by seed or root division. The flowers were traditionally collected on Saint John's Day (hence its name), June 24. It was then soaked in olive oil a few days, which turns the oil a surprising, bright red color. This was used as an anointing oil called blood of Christ.

To make a tonic tea, add 4 fresh leaves or a pinch of the dried herb to 1 cup of boiling water. Steep 15 minutes and strain. Drink only up to 2 cups per day for no longer than a week.

## AVAILABILITY
St.-John's-wort can be easily grown. The dried herb can be purchased at some herb or health food shops.

# Combining Herbs in Healing Tonics

We have already discussed fifty-three useful tonic herbs and their properties and effects on the body. Since each herb has different attributes and healing abilities, why not combine them into a multiingredient brew? A combination brew is easier to consume. We do not have to drink three or four different teas a day for several different problems, just one.

However, DO NOT use tonics as a replacement for medical advice. Herbal tonics can never replace competent medical diagnosis, but they can serve as helpful additions to treatments considered. Also, many open-minded physicians find information about herbs useful in their continuing search for appropriate and effective healing aids.

Two famous brews have revived interest in growing healing herbs. These brews have fascinating histories and have caused controversy because of the claims of thousands who have taken them. Reportedly, these drinks cure cancer and serious illnesses. So, it's important to learn a little about them before we begin to combine herbs into tonics for our own special uses.

## THE TALE OF ESSIAC

In the early 1920s an elderly Canadian woman was diagnosed with breast cancer; the recommended treatment was a mastectomy. Of course, the woman needed someone to talk to about her problem; so, she went to her neighbor, who was of Ojibwa (Chippewa) descent. When the neighbor learned of the woman's illness, she went to her cupboard and began mixing several different packages of dried herbs and set her teakettle to boil. She gave the resulting tea to the elderly woman to drink with instructions for brewing it herself. Within a short time, the woman found she was healed.

The old woman related this tale to a nurse who wanted the recipe, which she gave her. It's thought that the nurse modified the recipe somewhat. The nurse, whose name was Rene Caisse, christened her "improved" brew Essiac (*Caisse* spelled backwards). Caisse first tried the recipe on her aunt, who had inoperable stomach cancer with the liver also affected. Within 2 years, to Caisse's amazement, the aunt fully recovered; so, Caisse began using the formula on other terminal cancer patients. Fame of her success spread, and in 1938 a bill was introduced in the United States to legalize Essiac treatments. But the bill failed. The nurse's biggest fear was that the simple recipe would be revealed and possibly misused or that people with money would exploit it.

Eventually, the Resperin Corporation persuaded her to hand over the formula for a dollar in 1977. In December 1978 she died at age 90, and her dream of Essiac becoming recognized as a cancer treatment backed by research was never realized. Apparently, Resperin has had difficulty persuading physicians to cooperate in research.

In any case, one of Caisse's patients is thought to have gotten her hands on the recipe, because it has been circulating. Some people who have found the recipe mixed it up to sell to the general public. But it's so easy to make Essiac yourself, and that way you can control the quality of the ingredients. Common rhubarb was originally used in place of turkey rhubarb. Here's a version of the recipe.

## ESSIAC TONIC

*1 ounce of turkey rhubarb root* (Rheum palmatum) •
6½ cups of burdock root (Arctium lappa), *cut* •
½ *cup of slippery elm inner bark* (Ulmus rubra), *powdered* •
*1 pound of sheep sorrel* (Rumex acetosella), *powered*

Mix all the dried ingredients together. Add ¼ cup of this mixture to 2 quarts of boiling water. Use a deep pot and the purest water available. Cover and let boil 10 minutes Take off the heat, stir, cover again, and let steep for about 12 hours. Bring to a boil once again (15 to 20 minutes), strain, and bottle in sterilized containers. Refrigerate. To use, shake the bottle, and measure out 4 tablespoons of Essiac, added to ½ teacup of hot water. Add honey for sweetener, if you wish. Drink this every evening before bedtime on an empty stomach (2 to 3 hours after meals). No preservative has been used; so, if mold develops, discard that batch and make another.

Although Essiac has been hailed as a cancer cure, it does not have a 100 percent cure rate. Herbalists, like many medical practitioners, have been quick to acknowledge that no medicine is ever 100 percent effective, since it depends upon the circumstances and the individual patient. Essiac has been noted for healing many other chronic and degenerative conditions, particularly because of its blood-cleansing and immune-system strengthening ingredients. Slippery elm bark is a regenerative herb, sheep sorrel is a strengthener, and burdock is a strong blood cleanser, as is turkey rhubarb. These ingredients work together to help the body heal itself.

# HOXSEY'S DREAM

Another exciting formula thought capable of ending the misery of people afflicted with cancer and terminal illnesses was Hoxsey's Cure. Harry Hoxsey, with no medical training, a love of people and hatred of the American Medical Association, battled the medical establishment with no success.

But the discovery was really that of his grandfather, Dr. John Hoxsey, a veterinarian in the American Midwest. In the 1840s, the grandfather had diagnosed cancer in one of his horses, and with resignation put the horse out to pasture and waited for him to die. To the veterinarian's amazement, the horse did not die. In fact, the horse began to show signs of complete recovery. How could that be, he surely wondered. John Hoxsey placed food out for the horse, but the horse would not eat it. He then feared the horse would die of starvation. And so the veterinarian began watching the horse and observed that the horse was foraging and eating herbs it normally would not eat. Grandfather Hoxsey went out and gathered all the herbs the horse favored and created the Hoxsey formula, a liquid elixir containing ten tonic herbs.

The recipe was passed to family and friends until grandson Harry Hoxsey received it from his father on his deathbed. It is said that Harry promised his father to spread news of the elixir and to offer it free to people who could not afford it. In 1924 Harry Hoxsey opened a clinic in Taylorville, Illinois, and people came from around the country. The formula seemed to work; thousands claimed to be cured. And so, a war between the natural health community and the modern, mainstream, health community began.

The American Medical Association, which opposed Harry Hoxsey, was founded in part to make the medical profession a profitable venture. The organization has been instrumental in transforming medicine into an industry. Hoxsey, it seems, threatened the growing industry. He was perhaps considered a country bumpkin mixing up herbs which anyone could gather, and he appeared to be curing cancer and other serious illnesses, often without charging for services.

Although Harry Hoxsey was harassed and arrested for practicing medicine without a license, many tormentors eventually became supporters after they witnessed his seemingly miraculous cures for themselves. Whenever Hoxsey was arrested, his patients bailed him out or testified about the effectiveness of the formula.

Exasperated, the U.S. Food & Drug Administration (FDA) attempted to put Hoxsey and his clinics out of business. A law had been passed that required all medicines to contain only U.S. FDA-approved ingredients. None of the herbs in Hoxsey's formula were approved by the FDA; so, Hoxsey had violated federal law by offering the herbal tonic even if he did offer it free. In 1963 his clinics were closed, and Hoxsey's nurse, a former nonbeliever who had changed her mind after her mother had been cured of cancer, fled to Mexico to open a cancer clinic safe from attack. In the early 1970s, Hoxsey died of heart and liver failure. Many claim he died of a broken heart.

The formula for Hoxsey's Cure has been kept well guarded. I was unable to find out the amounts or the directions for preparing the brew. I did discover that it contained ten different herbs. Among them were burdock (*Rheum palmatum*), red clover, licorice root, barberry root, buckthorn (*Rhamnus frangula*), cascara sagrada (*Rhamnus purshiana*), prickly ash (*Zanthoxylum americanum*), stillingia root (*Stillingia sylvatica*), and two more dangerous herbs, poke root (*Phytolacca americana*, which is poisonous) and bloodroot (*Sanguinaria canadensis*).

Nine of these herbs inhibit tumors and behave as antiseptics as well. Five are antioxidants, a quality researchers believe may be key to preventing and possibly treating cancers. I'm not very familiar with a few of these herbs, but I've discovered in my research that all herbs used in this formula are strong alteratives. My main interest focused on poke and bloodroot. Both herbs are HIGHLY TOXIC with the wrong dosage, and since I don't know the correct dosages for Hoxsey's Cure, I'll highlight what I found out about these two herbs.

**POKE** (Toxic: CAN CAUSE DEATH) Native North American tribes in what are now the eastern United States and southeastern Canada used this root in poultices to treat tumors and skin eruptions. They passed on this medicinal use to early American Colonists. I've heard of folk healers placing a paste of poke root on a breast tumor. The skin disintegrates and allows the folk healer to lift out the tumor. This herb is an alterative and powerful purgative. The young spring leaves and shoots are cooked (although it is boiled twice to leach out toxic properties) and eaten as a spring green by old-timers. Research has found it to be a potent immune stimulant in correct dosages, and the leaf has been found to contain an antiviral protein similar to interferon, having antitumor properties. In the old herbal *The People's Common Sense Medical Adviser* (1866), R. V. Pierce, M.D., mentions using poke as an alterative herb in a decoction with the very conservative dosage of 3 to 10 drops.

**BLOODROOT** (Toxic: CAN CAUSE DEATH) Other North American tribes used bloodroot in teas for fevers and rheumatism. Tribes living near Lake Superior were known to have used the sap to cure skin cancers, and it was listed in the *U.S. Pharmacopoeia* until 1926. Bloodroot is an expectorant, useful for lung disorders and pneumonia. There are indications that it is good for cancer treatments, particularly skin cancer. Studies indicate that it is useful for breast cancer and superficial tumors. The dried rhizomes are used, but again, dosage is tricky and it is best not to experiment with the herb if you are not a qualified physician.

Leave these two herbs—poke and bloodroot—out of Hoxsey's formula if you wish to try it. One herbalist suggested you could add equal amounts of Hoxsey's herbs (minus poke and bloodroot), and mix well. Then add 4 to 6 tablespoons of the mixture per quart of water, bring it to a boil, and simmer 25 minutes. Cool and strain. Then add 1 to 3 tablespoons of this extract to 1 cup of hot water and drink each day.

As for the other herbs reportedly in the formula, buckthorn is a powerful purgative, and cascara sagrada, also called wahoo or sacred bark, was often an ingredient in tonics popular in the mid-1800s (made into a laxative tea by soaking the bark in water overnight and drinking it the next morning). Prickly ash was a general stimulant used in treating alcoholism. Stillingia is an expectorant and alterative. Other herbs included in this formula were discussed in previous chapters. Licorice root and burdock are powerful blood cleansers, and barberry and red clover are renewing herbs.

## MORE RECIPES HANDED DOWN

As you can see, many herbs can be blended together to help heal. Let's consider other tonic recipes handed down to us. Four Thieves' Vinegar was used during the late Middle Ages to protect against the plague. We can pick the recipe apart to see how they accomplished this goal. Here's one version of the recipe that leaves out two toxic ingredients.

### PLAGUE RELIEF or
### FOUR THIEVES' VINEGAR

*1 gallon of wine vinegar • 1 teaspoon of ground cloves •
4 ounces of sliced garlic • 4 ounces of sage leaves and flowers •
4 ounces of rosemary sprigs • 4 ounces of lavender flowers*

Combine, let stand 1 to 2 weeks, strain, and drink 1 cup daily.

The thieves wanted to avoid the plague, and we know today that the Black Death, a highly infectious disease, was caused by a bacterium (*Pasteurella pestis*) carried by fleas on rodents. It reduced Europe's population in the mid-14th century by nearly half. Symptoms included enlarged lymph nodes, septicemia with fever, prostration, and coma. Plague pneumonia was particularly severe; death was common.

Modern treatments for the plague include antibiotics and disinfection. How did the vinegar prove so effective? Four Thieves' Vinegar contains one of the most powerful natural antibiotics known: garlic, which discourages bacteria and viruses. Sage is highly antiseptic and acts as a strengthener. Rosemary fights bacterial and fungal infections, strengthening the body, and lavender has both stimulant and antiseptic properties. Mixed together, these herbs allowed the thieves to resist the plague. They were lucky to stumble upon the best recipe they could for keeping their bodies strong and destroying this deadly bacterium.

During the later tonic making and selling boom, the recorded recipes can help us understand the reasoning behind blending these herbs. One famous tonic, Dr. Pierce's Golden Medical Discovery or Alterative Extract, was thought highly nutritive and a good tonic, since it combined the best alteratives then known. It was made up mostly of queen's root, stone root, cherry bark, bloodroot, sacred bark, Oregon grape root, and glycerine.

Doctors and herbalists at that time agreed, as we do today, that all these herbs were tonic in nature. Queen's root, also known as stillingia, is an alterative which acts as a blood purifier. Stone root (*Collinsonia canadensis*) was regarded as an alterative, tonic, and stimulant. Cherry bark (*Prunus virginiana*) was deemed an excellent stomach tonic, especially good for the bronchial system and a sedative as well. Bloodroot's main therapeutic use was for pneumonia, asthma, bronchitis, and the respiratory system in general, although we could substitute safer tonic herbs today (see caution on p. 135). Sacred bark worked as a tonic for the intestines and the sympathetic nervous system. Oregon grape root is a strong tonic as well that acts on the lymphatic system.

In an old herbal, *The People's Common Sense Medical Advisor* (1918), published by the World's Dispensary Medical Association, Dr. R. V. Pierce states, "We are apt sometimes to overlook or set aside old, reliable remedies . . . for things of less medicinal value which are of more recent introduction to the attention of the medical profession."

Dr. Ayer of Massachusetts, who produced Ayer's Wild Cherry Expectorant, claimed that the tonic could cure catarrh, bronchitis, and influenza. He freely published the recipe for the general public. It included 2 fluid drams of tincture of bloodroot; 3 fluid drams each of antimonial wine, ipecac wine, and syrup of wild cherry bark; and 3 grains of acetate of morphia. Of course, the morphine helped take away the pain, as did the addition of wines, but bloodroot is tonic in nature, with expectorant properties and generally helpful for the respiratory system. Wild cherry bark is an expectorant, too, which helps break up congestion. So this tonic, although it contained addictive morphine, alcohol, and bloodroot, had healing properties and would have worked quite effectively without dangerous or addictive additions. It would not have had immediate and noticeable effects, as the original recipe did, but it would work as tonics do, slowly but surely.

Let's look at two more recipes from the past to see if we can guess their usage. Here's a version of the recipe for Stoughton Tonic Bitters.

## STOUGHTON TONIC BITTERS

*6 ounces of orange peel, powdered •*
*½ ounce of American saffron, powdered •*
*1½ ounces of Virginia snakeroot, powdered •*
*8 ounces of gentian root, powdered •*
*4 pints of water • 4 pints of alcohol*

Mix and let set for 14 days. Strain, adding enough diluted alcohol to make 1 gallon.

The water and alcohol are merely the media which extract the healing properties of the tonic herbs. The orange peel, which I thought at first was a flavoring, turns out to be a digestive. So, what remains are American saffron, Virginia snakeroot, and gentian. Saffron has been traditionally advised for insomnia, colds, tumors, cancer, and as an appetite stimulant. Virginia snakeroot (*Aristolochia serpentaria*) is a bitter stimulant tonic, helpful especially when combined with other, more powerful, bitters. And gentian is an extremely bitter herb that stimulates the digestive tract.

All these herbs have been used for stimulating digestion, which suggests that this tonic would be helpful for anorexia. Stoughton Tonic Bitters may also be helpful for elderly people who have lost their appetite, people with poor circulation, or people recovering from an illness.

The second recipe comes from the Shakers and was created by Thomas Corbett. It became the most well-known of over thirty types of medicines developed and sold by the Shaker Canterbury community in New Hampshire. It was simply called Syrup of Sarsaparilla. Since this tonic was intended for large-scale sales, the amounts of herbs used in the original recipe were enormous: 100 pounds of sarsaparilla root and so on. The herbs in this syrup, in order of greatest quantity, were sarsaparilla, dandelion, yellow dock, mandrake (or ginseng), black cohosh, garget, Indian hemp, and juniper berries.

These herbs indicate that Syrup of Sarsaparilla would be a powerful blood cleanser, since sarsaparilla, dandelion, and yellow dock are included. Other special attributes are that yellow dock is a good laxative; sarsaparilla has antibiotic properties, gets rid of wastes, and is helpful for the lymphatic and circulatory systems; and dandelion is highly nutritive. Dandelion is also helpful for liver and skin disorders. It is a diuretic, helps stimulate and strengthen the body, and can be helpful to people who are overweight.

Ginseng helps renew weakened bodies suffering from long-standing illnesses, and black cohosh is a renewing tonic herb. Since it was widely popular, the Shakers were able to document the many varied illnesses this tonic helped. Among them were chronic inflammations of the digestive system, rheumatism, liver disorders, skin eruptions, asthma, dropsy, tuberculosis, dysentery, diarrhea, ailments arising from blood impurities, and female complaints.

## CREATING YOUR OWN BLENDS

So now we're ready to mix our own healing tonics according to our specific needs. What are those needs? Well, perhaps you're run-down and you're suffering with arthritis. For you, blood-cleansing herbs are the ones you should focus on first. Suppose you want to prevent illness and build up your immune system to tip-top health because you've been under a lot of stress. Then you'd blend strengthening tonic herbs to build the immune system, energizers, and renewing tonic herbs to ease stress and tension. Each person is likely to have specific and varied symptoms and problems. Since the herbs are varied and have many capabilities, you'll be sure to find the tonic blend best for you if you take time to review the many herbs described in these chapters. Make notes of the different herbs you know have an affinity for healing the problems you have. It's important to balance your blend so that it can accomplish many different tasks in one dose.

When I do this, I first identify my main problem and then any secondary problems. Let's say you have a problem with gout, but you're also overweight and have high blood pressure. The principal problem is high blood pressure since it's more serious, but you also have gout and excess weight to contend with. Which herbs will help you out?

## HEART-STRENGTHENING GOUT TONIC

*hawthorn berries • dandelion root • chamomile •*
*cayenne pepper • stinging nettle • apple pectin • ginseng*

Would you have chosen these herbs? Let's do another. Suppose you are suffering from chronic Epstein-Barr syndrome and you're also prone to herpes outbreaks. Stress brings on attacks in both illnesses; so, we would include herbs to counter stress (like catnip, barberry, or valerian) along with immune-system strengtheners (like echinacea or goldenseal), as well as blood-purifying, energizing, and one of two alterative tonic herbs.

What follows are some recipes for various illnesses. You can use these, or change them according to your preferences.

# ARTHRITIS TONIC

*1 tablespoon of black cohosh root, powdered •*
*1 tablespoon of chopped garlic • 1 tablespoon of skullcap •*
*1 tablespoon of comfrey • 1 teaspoon of cayenne pepper •*
*1 teaspoon of parsley • 1 quart of vinegar*

Cover all these herbs with the vinegar. Let sit in sun for 2 weeks to make a tincture, and strain. Add 1 tablespoon of the mixture to 1 cup of boiling water. Drink this cup slowly in sips throughout the day.

Cayenne pepper, a member of the nightshade family (like potatoes, tomatoes, and other peppers), can irritate those sensitive to solanine (estimated to be as much as 10 percent of the population), which creates an enzyme that irritates joints. Here cayenne is used as a catalyst.

# MIGRAINE TONIC

*1 tablespoon of hop • 1 tablespoon of peppermint •*
*1 tablespoon of chamomile • 1 tablespoon of violet • 1 quart of vodka*

Mix herbs well and add to the vodka. Let steep 2 weeks in a sunny window and strain. Add 1 teaspoon to 1 cup of boiling water.

# COLD, SINUS, AND FLU TONIC

*1 teaspoon of ginseng, powdered • 3 tablespoons of rose hips •*
*1 tablespoon of garlic, chopped • 1 tablespoon of catnip •*
*1 teaspoon of cayenne pepper • 1 quart of vodka*

Mix herbs well and add to the vodka. Let steep 2 weeks in a sunny window and strain. Add 1 teaspoon to 1 cup of boiling water. Let cool to lukewarm. Drink up to 3 cups per day.

### Specific How-To's

Blended tonics are the easiest to make when you prepare a tincture of the different herbs with a 90-proof vodka or gin or with a good quality of apple cider vinegar. This solution extracts all the phytochemicals from the plants (in a concentrated form), making it easy to store and use (less space is taken up). And your tonic will be well preserved.

The basic method for making a tincture is really very simple. Use 6 to 8 tablespoons of herb per quart of vodka or vinegar. You can vary the amounts of each herb to make up the 6 to 8 tablespoons, but a rule of thumb is 3 parts of one herb (using a specially chosen herb for the main or most severe problem) and 1 part of three herbs that follow it (for secondary problems). Set this mixture, strained and bottled, in a sunny window for 14 days. Use 1 tablespoon of the mixture per day in hot water (spacing dosage as necessary through the day). Since 1 tablespoon is equal to 3 teaspoons, you can drink up to 3 cups a day adding 1 teaspoon to each.

This isn't a strict method, though. In A *Compendium of Modern Pharmacy and Druggists' Formulary* (1881), Walter B. Kilner describes a formula called Simpler's Method of Making Tinctures. This involved covering the herbs with warmed alcohol or vinegar (making sure the liquid covered the herbs with 2-inch head room). Then the mixture was placed in a sunny window for 4 weeks and strained. Rebottled, the mixture was stored in a dark cupboard and the dosage taken in hot water or added to juice. Another method was for every ounce of fresh or dried herb, add 4 ounces of alcohol (or 2 ounces of water and 2 ounces of alcohol). Let the mixture stand up to 14 days and strain. As you can see, amounts and times of steeping can vary. You have to remember, though, that the longer the mixture steeps and the greater the quantity of herbs used, the stronger the tincture. So, you'll need less of the tincture; remember, it's concentrated. It's best, therefore, to stick as closely as possible to the basic formula.

How long should you take a tonic? No medicine should be used on a continuous basis. Take it until the symptoms are gone and you feel healthy again. Most herbalists agree that tonics designed for more serious illnesses can be taken up to 6 to 8 weeks, with a resting period between, and then resumed as needed.

## METRIC EQUIVALENTS

| | |
|---|---|
| 1 inch = 2.54 centimeters | 1 millimeter = 0.039 inch |
| 1 foot - 30.5 centimeters | 1 meter = 3.28 feet |
| 1 cup = 0.24 liter | 1 liter = 2.1 pints = 1.06 quarts |
| 1 tablespoon = 15 milliliters | 1 pound = 0.45 kilograms |
| 1 teaspoon = 5 milliliters | 1 ounce = 28 grams |
| 1 pint = 0.48 liter | 1 8-ounce glass = 1 cup or 0.24 liters |
| 1 quart = 0.96 liter | 1 gallon = 3.84 liters |

**To Convert Fahrenheit to Centigrade**

$$(F \text{ degrees} - 32) \, 5/9 = C \text{ degrees}$$

# Index

⤖